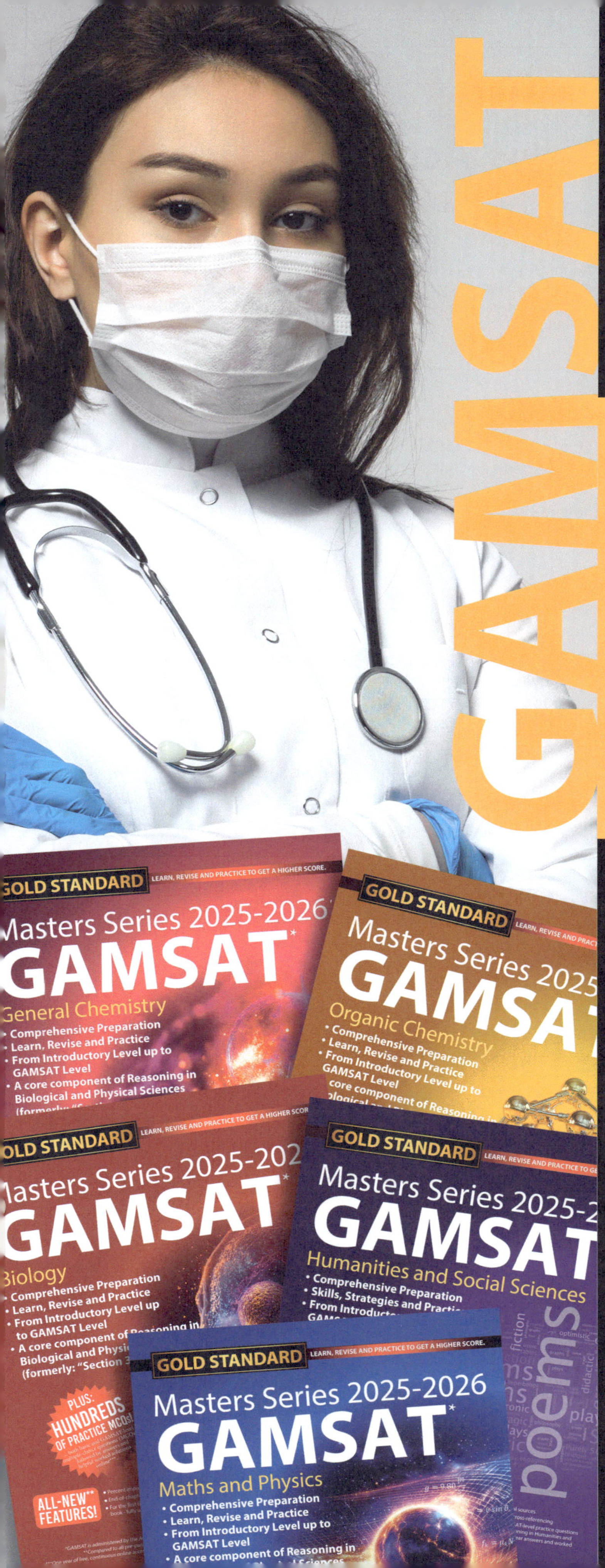

GOLD STANDARD

PERMISSION GRANTED

If you wish to share your study experience in social media (e.g. Instagram, TikTok, YouTube, etc.), Gold Standard GAMSAT gives you the permission to include any of our books (cover and/or interior pages, though never all pages from a chapter), and/or short segments of our videos, in your content. Share your study journey and inspire others!

01 **Editor and Author**
Brett Ferdinand BSc MD-CM

02 **Contributors**
Lisa Ferdinand BA MA
Sean Pierre BSc MD
Kristin Finkenzeller BSc MD
Ibrahima Diouf BSc MSc PhD
Charles Haccoun BSc MD-CM
Timothy Ruger BA MA
Jeanne Tan Te

03 **Illustrators**
Harvie W. Gallatiera BS CompE
Gilbert Rafanan BSc

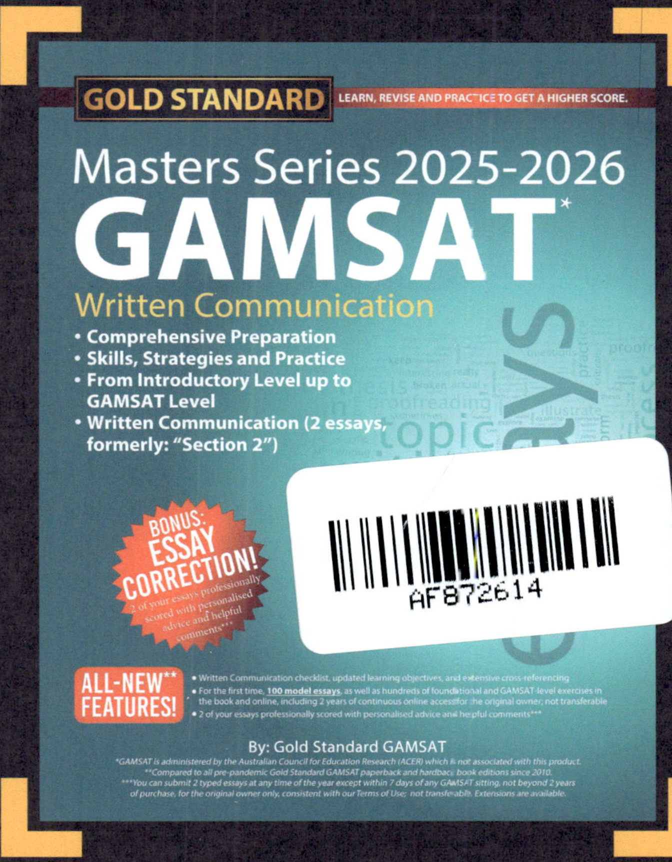

Register your book!

Free Online Access*

Additional Written Communication exercises + two of your essays professionally scored with personalised advice and helpful comments.**

*Two years of continuous access for the original owner of this textbook upon online registration at www.gamsat-prep.com/gamsat-essays-written-communication/
**You can submit 2 typed essays at any time of the year except within 7 days of any GAMSAT sitting.

Please note: Benefits last for two years from the date of online registration, for the original book owner only, and are not transferable; unauthorized access and use outside the Terms of Use posted on GAMSAT-prep.com may result in account deletion; if you are not the original owner, you can purchase your virtual access card separately at GAMSAT-prep.com.

Online access reduces digital piracy, allows the addition of relevant multimedia, permits more detailed worked solutions, reduces the retail price, and saves trees!

ISBN 978-1-927338-89-6

Address all inquiries, comments, or suggestions to the publisher. For Terms of Use go to: www.GAMSAT-prep.com

Gold Standard GAMSAT Product Contact Information

Distribution in Australia, NZ, Asia

Woodslane Pty Ltd 10 Apollo Street
Warriewood NSW 2102 Australia
ABN: 76 003 677 549
learn@gamsat-prep.com

Distribution in Europe

Central Books 99 Wallis
Road LONDON,
E9 5LN, United Kingdom
orders@centralbooks.com

Distribution in North America

RuveneCo Publishing
334 Cornelia Street #559
Plattsburgh, New York 12901, USA
buy@gamsatbooks.com

GAMSAT (Graduate Medical School Admissions Test)

Computer-based exam held at test centres internationally for graduate-entry medicine

Written Communication (Writing Tasks A & B)

- formerly "Section 2"

2 essays responding to 2 different themes using sound reasoning and competent English-writing skills (essays must be typed)

Writing Task A: sociocultural theme (e.g., free speech, justice, social media)
Writing Task B: personal-social themes (e.g., humour, love, happiness)

Reasoning in Humanities and Social Sciences

- formerly "Section 1"

multiple-choice section with stimulus materials requiring comprehension and analysis of non-science content

poetry • proverbs cartoons • novels or play excerpts • travel and/or medical journal entries • social science graphs

Reasoning in Biological and Physical Sciences

- formerly "Section 3"

multiple-choice section with questions mostly based on science passages that require problem-solving and graph analysis

first-year undergraduate level Biology (40%), General Chemistry (20%) & Organic Chemistry (20%) • A-level/Leaving Certificate/ Year 12 level Physics (20%)

Top GAMSAT Score: 100
Average GAMSAT Score: 57

Summary of the new Digital-format GAMSAT Exam Day

	KEY POINTS	EVENT	DURATION
Written Communication	Produce ideas in writing with clarity and soundness; essays are typed with no copy/paste function	2 essays typed on a computer (for all sections including the essays: no longer is there a formal, dedicated reading time)	65 minutes
Arrival and Sitting of Exam	Bring only the acceptable ID documents and permitted items to the test centre as specified in ACER's GAMSAT Information Booklet	Security, identification, health protocols	15-45 minutes
Reasoning in Humanities and Social Sciences	Key skills are reading speed and comprehension of information within socio-cultural contexts	62 MCQs* (the test centre will provide you with 2 sheets of A4 scratch paper; *option*: whiteboard)	100 minutes
Break	Consider packing your own lunch to avoid queues with nervous chatter	–	20 minutes
Reasoning in Biological and Physical Sciences	Analyse and solve problems: 40% Biology, 40% Chemistry (equally split between General and Organic); 20% Physics	75 MCQs* (the test centre will provide you with 2 new sheets of A4 scratch paper; *option*: whiteboard)	150 minutes
Total Test Time	Success requires stamina; stamina improves with practice.	–	5 hours, 15 minutes

*MCQs: multiple-choice questions, 4 options per question with only 1 best answer. Note that the 'old' GAMSAT had a dedicated 'reading time' of 10 minutes for each of Section 1 and 3, and 5 minutes for Section 2. During that reading time, students were not permitted to write or mark their exam paper in any way. The new digital GAMSAT has added time for each of the 3 exam sections as a legacy to 'reading time'; however, in practice, you can use your exam time in any way that you see fit.

**It might be a good idea to allocate a whole day to sit the GAMSAT test to allow for any contingencies and/or technical issues that you might encounter. Safety measures and health protocols should be carefully anticipated when making travel arrangements and accommodations to and from the testing centre.

Common formula for acceptance:

GPA + GAMSAT score + Interview = Medical School Admissions

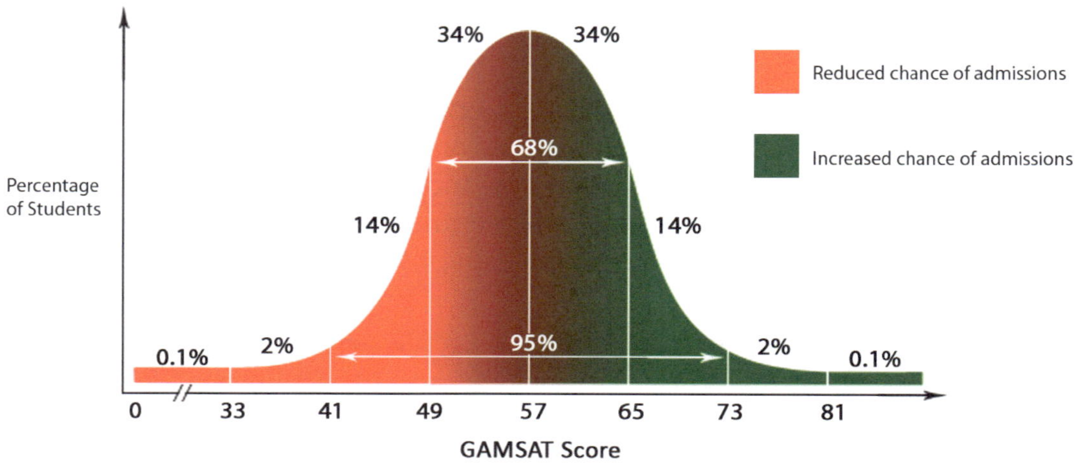

Typical Overall GAMSAT Score Distribution (Approx)

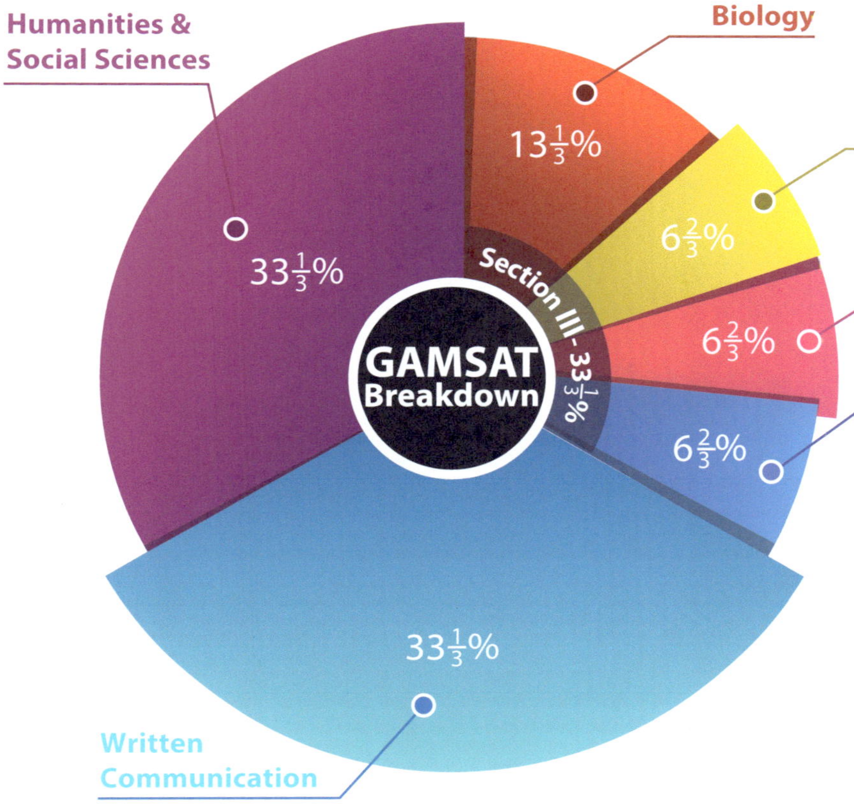

Please note: Some medical schools weigh all 3 sections equally, as illustrated in the pie chart to the left, while others weigh Section III (the sciences) twice as seen below.

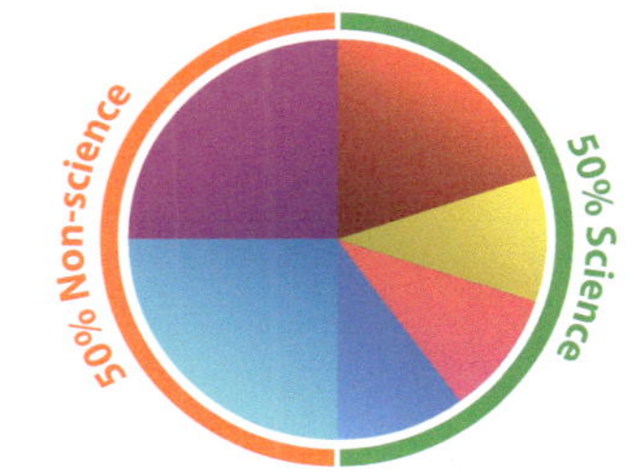

GAMSAT is challenging, get organised.

gamsat-prep.com/free-GAMSAT-study-schedule

1. How to study

- Learn, revise and practice using the GAMSAT Masters Series book(s) and/or videos.
- Complete all exercises and multiple-choice practice questions in this book.
- Consolidate: create and study from your personal summaries (= Gold Notes) daily. Create study cards or audio files from your Gold Notes to increase your study efficiency.

2. Once you have completed your studies

- Sit a full-length GAMSAT practice test.
- Analyse mistakes and all worked solutions.
- Consolidate: Revise all your Gold Notes and create more.

3. Sit multiple mock exams

- ACER GAMSAT practice exams with free Gold Standard worked solutions on YouTube
- Free full-length Gold Standard (GS) mock exam GS-Free with helpful, detailed worked solutions
- HEAPS: 15 full-length exams, 5 in the book and 10 online with the new, digital GAMSAT format

4. How much time do you need to study?

- On average, 3-6 hours per day for 3-6 months; depending on life experiences, 2 weeks may be enough and 8 months could be insufficient.
- Try to study full on for 1-2 weeks and then adjust your expectations for your personal, ideal study time.

5. Recommended GAMSAT Communities

- All countries (mainly Australia): pagingdr.net
- Mainly the UK: thestudentroom.co.uk (Medicine Community Discussion)
- Mainly Ireland: boards.ie (GAMSAT and GEM forum)

Is there something in the Masters Series that you did not understand? Don't get frustrated, get online:

gamsat-prep.com/forum

Table of Contents

Note that: H = High-level Importance; M = Medium-level Importance; L = Low-level Importance.

INTRODUCTION

> *"Read a thousand books, and your words will flow like a river."*
> — Lisa See

A chorus of clickety-clackety, clickety-clack may greet your ears during your real digital GAMSAT experience. Some candidates will release a tornado of creativity, and others, pure unintelligible refuse. Fortunately, since 2024, you can type your real exam essays at a secure location that you can choose (e.g., your home) so that the only clickety-clackety sounds should originate from your digits!

The purpose of GAMSAT Written Communication (WC, 2 essays), ACER says, is to assess your ability "to organise and express your thoughts in a logical and effective way," of course, in writing. Starting in 2020, *writing* began to signify *typing*. That was the year GAMSAT was forced to quickly shift from paper with a writing implement, to a computer with a keyboard, due to the global pandemic. Though you will type your essays, you are permitted to use some old-fashioned A4 sheets of scratch (*note* or *scrap*) paper to help you plan your essay. As an alternative, ACER gives you the option to use an erasable whiteboard to plan your essay or, more generally, for notetaking.

> *"Write. Rewrite. When not writing or rewriting, read. I know of no shortcuts."*
> —Larry L. King, WD

In this Masters Series textbook, we will examine creative ideas to optimise your GAMSAT Written Communication score. We hope to help you further develop your language skills and explore essay-writing techniques and strategies. You will learn the operating procedure to develop a conservative (safe) essay structure vs. a more risqué, creative composition with its many pros and cons.

You will have the opportunity to practice until you develop your own style. You will also be able to read more than 100 model essays (WC 5.1, Gold Ideas). You can observe the mental gymnastics involved and note the rewards and penalties. In the prelude to the model essays presented in Gold Ideas, we will remind you that ACER assesses essay responses for plagiarism: forewarned is forearmed.

And then, what follows is the *sine qua non* of this textbook, where we hope you will apply '*sine qua non*' in context: GAMSAT Written Communication, essay writing. Two of your masterpieces will be professionally corrected and returned to you with specific comments and guidance* ('legalese' down below).

> *"And by the way, everything in life is writable about if you have the outgoing guts to do it, and the imagination to improvise. The worst enemy to creativity is self-doubt."*
> — Sylvia Plath

Our essay-correction team has dozens of years of experience and you will find the critique given for your essays both helpful and specific. The experience on our team and feedback from successful students produced a system of categorisation of some pages in this book according to their level of importance. It is not a scientific process but you might find it to be a helpful hand.

Writing an essay is not a spectator sport. This book is filled with exercises and practice questions to keep you engaged, and most importantly, to get you in touch with your inner writer.

Let's begin!

– BF, MD

*You can submit 2 typed essays at any time of the year except within 7 days of any GAMSAT sitting, not beyond 2 years of purchase, for the original owner only, consistent with our Terms of Use; not transferable. Proof of purchase may be required. Register at: www.gamsat-prep.com/gamsat-essays-written-communication/.

GAMSAT-Prep.com

WRITTEN COMMUNICATION

PREPARATION FOR GAMSAT WRITTEN COMMUNICATION (ESSAYS)

4.1 Overview

GAMSAT Written Communication (WC) is comprised of 2 writing tasks, which should be completed within a 65-minute time limit (the new, digital GAMSAT timing). Each writing task has four or five quotations - listed as "Comments" - that appertain to a common theme.

Historically, candidates were given 5 minutes to read through the instructions and quotations before the actual test would begin. It was forbidden to write or make any notes during the 5 minutes of reading time. Reading time *per se*, as it existed before 2020, is no longer. The 5 minutes has been added to the traditional 60 minutes, but to be clear, you can begin writing the moment the 65-minute timer starts.

Why write an essay?

In the early 1990s, the essay was included in the American MCAT exam following complaints from the deans of various medical schools concerning the communication skills of medical students. Subsequently, it was included in the inaugural GAMSAT in 1995 and, of course, has continued to this day. Ironically, the new MCAT no longer has an essay section.

GAMSAT WC will measure your ability to:

1) articulate your perspective on a given topic;
2) synthesise ideas and concepts;
3) express ideas in a logical and cohesive way;
4) write clearly, using standard English and appropriate grammar, spelling and punctuation.

Written Communication is the only GAMSAT section which is not multiple choice. Students must type two essays in response to two different themes. The first essay "Task A" is supposed to address a socio-cultural theme and the second essay "Task B", personal and social themes. You may use 1 or more of the given quotations as the basis for your written response. In selecting topics, ACER makes an effort to minimise factors which might disadvantage candidates from non-English speaking backgrounds.

You are not expected to write a short, polished essay of final draft quality. The people grading your exam are aware that you only had 65 minutes to write two essays. Nevertheless, you will be expected to come up with a 'good' essay expressing your well-considered view of the ideas or themes presented in each writing task. Please refer to WC 4.7 for a scoring key. You may also consult WC 4.8 and GAMSAT-prep.com for examples of what a 'good' essay is in the eyes of the markers.

Several years ago, ACER suggested a different writing format of response to the socio-political theme of Task A as compared to the personal theme of Task B. However, in recent years, no mention of a particular essay style has been made in any of ACER's official materials, and many candidates have scored well using the same writing style in both Tasks A and B. In fact, some candidates find it much easier to practice and follow one format.

Real GAMSAT Written Communication Topics Reported in Public Forums

YEAR	Writing Task A	Writing Task B
2020	• conspiracy theories; poverty; war • art; information; criminality; the future • social media/clicktivism; journalism	• food; passion; love; bullying • gender; altruism; cynicism • personality traits; family
2019	• population control/family size • authority • taxes	• role model • recreational activities • prejudice and intolerance
2018	• democracy • our changing society • superstition	• ambition • consumerism • freedom
2017	• state of politics and public fear • multiculturalism	• celebrity culture • past vs present
2016	• freedom of speech • experience vs knowledge	• pets / animals • dreams / fame
2015	• human nature • cooperation • government	• imagination / fantasy • self-identity
2014	• cultural diversity • modern communication and technology	• happiness • art and its impact on society
2013	• meritocracy • government • superstition vs science	• marriage • work / play • idleness / procrastination
2012	• nanny state • technology	• love • life goals
2011	• affirmative action • space exploration	• happiness • humour
2010	• censorship • political correctness	• self-confidence • competition
2009	• intelligence • the role of government	• age and wisdom • media and its impact on society
2008	• past, present, future • racism	• wisdom and knowledge • optimism
2007	• human nature • nationalism / identity	• humour • work

Note: Themes are usually different in the March and September sittings and, sometimes, in different testing locations. This explains the numerous themes in a single exam year.

Medium-level Importance

Of course, those who possess significant skills in prose should work to their strengths. A word of caution, though: personal essays can be difficult to control at times, and can attract the disapproval of essay markers if they become ill-structured or overly sentimental. In this case, using the more objective style of argumentative-persuasive would be a better option.

Either way, an organised structure and ideas that display sound reasoning, supported by relevant examples, are central to a high-scoring Written Communication typed response.

4.1.1 General Pointers for Written Communication

While you do not need any specific knowledge to do well in this section, you should read from varied sources (*see* RHSS 3.2.1) to familiarise yourself with current political and social concerns.

You are expected to write a first-draft quality essay. A few grammatical, punctuation or spelling errors will not affect your mark greatly. However, a large number of such errors to the extent that your ideas become difficult to follow will harm you. You are allowed to delete words, sentences or passages. Computer copy/paste is disabled. Do not try to recopy an entire essay from your scratch paper. You are unlikely to have sufficient time to do this.

A title is not mandated but it could be helpful especially if it were catchy or intriguing. A good title should grab the reader's attention and - having crystallised the essay's thesis - orient the reader to the literary feast that is about to unveil. Both tasks must have at least 3 paragraphs: an introduction, the body and the conclusion.

The use of creativity can be great. For example, some students choose to write the essay (especially Task A) as though it is a conversation between two people. Other students use metaphors. For example, you can use a video camera as a metaphor of an objective observer that switches from scene to scene. In the final scene (the conclusion or resolution), one could begin by saying: "And now, the camera is truly in focus" as one describes how the conflict is resolved.

Though such creative expressions can be quite powerful, they cannot make up for the following basic fact: you must address the needs of the essay. You must clearly deal with the concerns of ACER which includes: **(1)** addressing the central theme clearly; **(2)** applying at least one of the quotations to your essay; **(3)** demonstrating logical thinking; **(4)** communicating your ideas in a clear and organised manner; and to a lesser extent, **(5)** technical issues.

Of course, being "overly" creative could have its own risks (i.e. inappropriate distraction). Creativity is best left to those with significant literary ability. It is crucial that candidates become expert at their essay structure and develop a strong body of knowledge and arguments for GAMSAT-style issues. Without a practiced writing style, strong structure, and an eclectic body of knowledge, no amount of gloss or ingenuity will score well – markers will see your essays for the mere veneer they are.

For Writing Task A, since this is formal writing, minimise your use of contractions as well as first-person and second-person pronouns ("I," "me," "you"). For both tasks, consider avoiding using contracted words such as "can't", "don't" or "won't". Finally, attempt to expand your vocabulary by avoiding the use of negating prefixes such as 'not', 'in' or 'un'.

For example, instead of saying "not complete" use the positive form of the word, which is "partial". Another example might be using the word "vague" instead of 'unclear'. The use of positive terms will elevate the quality of your essay.

Specific examples can be powerful from history or from current affairs. Both will be greatly bolstered with the advice in Masters Series RHSS 3.2.1 and RHSS 3.2.2 - irrespective of your academic background.

SPOILER ALERT

Gold Standard has cross-referenced the content in this book to examples from ACER's official GAMSAT practice materials. It is for you to decide when you want to explore these questions since you may want to preserve some of ACER's materials for timed mock-exam practice.

The 'old' exam format is known to have recurring Written Communication themes coming up in the actual test. **Examples –** Education (WC-74); Free Speech (WC-79); Love (WC-83); and Work (WC-89). On the other hand, candidates who have sat the new digital exam format reported getting different themes and with a wider range of issues than in past sittings. Nevertheless, it is always a good idea to practise responding to as many themes as possible such as those found in the ACER practice tests. **Examples –** Technology (WC-75) Task A of 3; Government (WC-76) Task A of 4; Humour (WC-139) Task B of 1; Family (WC-148) Task B of 4. Note that the eBook (booklet) number 1 is ACER's *GAMSAT Practice Questions*; eBook number 3 is *GAMSAT Practice Test 1*; and eBook number 4 is *GAMSAT Practice Test 2*.

Written Communication Checklist

- ☐ Access your free online account at www.gamsat-prep.com/gamsat-essays-written-communication/ to view additional model essays, discussion boards and most importantly: to have 2 of your essays professionally corrected. Note that you can submit 2 typed essays at any time of the year except within 7 days of any GAMSAT sitting, not beyond 2 years of purchase, for the original owner only, consistent with our Terms of Use; not transferable. The average turnaround time is 1 week.
- ☐ Complete a maximum of 1 page of notes using symbols/abbreviations to represent the content for every 10-15 pages that you read in this book. These are your Gold Notes.
- ☐ Consider your options based on your optimal way of learning:
  - ☐ Create your own, tangible study cards or try the free app: Anki.
  - ☐ Record your voice reading your Gold Notes onto your smartphone (*memo*) and listen during exercise, transportation, etc.
  - ☐ Consider reading at least 1 source material every day (e.g., poems of a single author, a synopsis of a novel, an article from a scientific journal that caught your interest, etc.). Note down the main idea or ideas of the piece on your scratch paper. Determine or surmise the author's sentiment or purpose for writing the material.
- ☐ Reassess your schedule for your full-length GAMSAT practice tests: ACER and/or HEAPS exams. Schedule regular WC practice tests, ideally at the same time of day that you would be expected to sit your real GAMSAT. Consider using the personalised essay-correction service from Gold Standard, or using AI, while adding to your abbreviated Gold Notes.
- ☐ Reassess your progress in scheduling and/or evaluating stress reduction techniques such as regular exercise (sports), yoga, meditation and/or mindfulness exercises (*see* YouTube for suggestions).

4.2 Key Skills to Develop for Written Communication

A Written Communication response:
- must be relevant to the theme of the writing task
- must express a well-thought-out opinion
- must demonstrate sound reasoning
- must be supported by evidence
- must be well-structured

It must be noted that assessment in Written Communication largely focusses on a candidate's ability to form an educated opinion and validate it using logic and reason. In other words, you are to write about what you think, NOT how much knowledge you have, about the topic. The ideas that you will discuss must be highly relevant to what the quotations are talking about, and they must demonstrate careful reasoning. Your ideas must be supported by evidence. You cannot simply state an idea without detailing supporting examples and theory; or in the case of personal essays, relevant anecdotes. Keep in mind that your essay will not be marked for having the most correct idea but for having a logical point of view. Having said that, you must still keep in mind that a real person is marking your essay. Unsavoury or politically incorrect ideas may require a higher burden of proof. While remaining objective, generally distasteful ideas will likely have negative implications for how a person views your work.

Typically, the most interesting ideas will get the most marks.

4.2.1 Generating the Response

Forming a response for a Written Communication writing task starts with two important skills - identifying the theme and stating your thesis.

- Identifying the Theme

While you will be asked to generate a written response to one or more of the given quotations - referred in the exam as "comments" - a particular set will noticeably talk about a common topic. Some comments will offer contradicting views; hence, the theme is presented as a debatable issue. In other cases, the comments will convey varying definitions of the same subject.

Your initial task is to determine what the comments, when taken together, are trying to say about an idea. This is different from merely identifying the topic. Finding the theme means answering the question: "What is it about this topic that the comments are saying?"

Even if you choose to develop an essay based on just one or two comments, you still need to consider the general context within which an idea is discussed.

Still, some students make the mistake of either reacting to the topic alone or choosing one of the comments and discussing a point that may be true within the quotation's context but so far off from the main idea (i.e. the theme) of all the comments. Let's take the following as an example:

* * * * *

Comment 1

Justice is justly represented blind, because she sees no difference in the parties concerned.

William Penn

* * * * *

Comment 2

Justice cannot be for one side alone, but must be for both.

Eleanor Roosevelt

* * * * *

Comment 3

It is better that ten guilty persons escape than one innocent suffer.

William Blackstone

* * * * *

Comment 4

It is more important that innocence be protected than it is that guilt be punished, for guilt and crimes are so frequent in this world that they cannot all be punished.

John Adams

* * * * *

Comment 5

> Justice consists not in being neutral between right and wrong, but in finding out the right and upholding it, wherever found, against the wrong.
>
> Theodore Roosevelt

As an aside, it is recommended that you learn about important historical figures such as William Blackstone or Theodore Roosevelt. Although the recent GAMSATs have not credited the sources of their quotes in the stimulus, this has been common practice in the past. If you understand the biography of a famous figure, you are likely to have a better insight into his or her statement. In general, historical biographies are great repositories of ideas and can serve as evidence for your arguments.

Going back to our sample quotations, the word "justice" is mentioned repeatedly, so this must be the topic. Now here's an example of an incorrect response: you recognise that the topic of this writing task is justice, so you open your essay with another quote by Abraham Lincoln: "I have always found that mercy bears richer fruits than strict justice." Then you proceed to cite the arguments between strictly enforcing justice and balancing it with mercy.

Or, you pick the fourth comment and talk about how punishment can leave a negative mark on a person's life. Then you cite an example about a young offender who was sent to prison for shoplifting. While in prison, he was exposed to cruelty and violence. This traumatic experience became an impetus for him to resent the justice system and become a ruthless criminal.

While the discussion in both cases may be very interesting, the general topic of this writing task does not really pertain to justice vs mercy or crime and punishment, but to justice being nondiscriminatory. So how can you mine the five comments for a main idea?

Here is a good procedure that you can follow to determine a theme:

First, read all the comments and note the words or phrases that are often mentioned. Repetition of words and phrases means that these are being emphasised. In our example, the words "justice", "guilt" or "guilty" and "innocence" or "innocent" are mentioned the most.

Second, observe how each comment either discusses the repeated words in a positive or a negative light. Note that the comments highlight facets of meaning or aspects of a given topic.

The first two comments speak of justice as making no distinction between different parties or sides. The next two comments place more importance in the protection of the innocent rather than punishing the guilty. The last comment views justice as upholding what is right.

Third, synthesise the ideas from all the comments. This is what you should react to. Your essay will either support or contradict this idea in the comments.

Again from our example, we were able to sift three ideas: that justice does not discriminate between two parties; that justice can only be achieved if the innocent is protected; and justice should always seek for what is right. We can then phrase this as a debatable issue: Should justice remain impartial or should justice ensure that the innocent is protected and uphold what is right?

Now you can decide which side to take and defend. The stand you choose will help formulate your thesis statement.

Let's take another set of quotations and apply the three-step approach that we just discussed:

* * * * *

Comment 1

Parents are always more ambitious for their children than they are for themselves.

* * * * *

Comment 2

We never know the love of a parent till we become parents ourselves.
Henry Ward Beecher

* * * * *

Comment 3

Parents can only give good advice or put them on the right paths, but the final forming of a person's character lies in their own hands.
Anne Frank

* * * * *

Comment 4

Some mothers are kissing mothers and some are scolding mothers, but it is love just the same, and most mothers kiss and scold together.
Pearl S. Buck

Comment 5

> A father's goodness is higher than the mountain, a mother's goodness deeper than the sea.
>
> Japanese Proverb

First, the most repeated word in this writing task is "parents".

Second, the first comment says that parents want their children to have a better life or future than their own. The second comment says children will only appreciate their parents when they become one. The third comment says parents can only guide their children but their children will still decide for themselves. The last two comments basically express the same view - every parent shows his or her love in different ways.

Third, we are now aware that while there are four thoughts on "parents" in this writing task, they all have to do with how parents show love or provide guidance to their children. This should now become the backdrop of your essay's discussion.

You can choose to agree or disagree with the idea that no matter the parenting style, parents want what's best for their children. Alternatively, you can expound on the issue of parents being overprotective and whether or not this is justifiable. Whichever perspective you choose, it needs to be expressed in the form of a thesis statement.

- Stating the Thesis

Whether your essay takes the form of a discursive or a reflective piece, the thesis statement has to be apparent. The thesis statement serves as your main response because it embodies the overall point of your essay. It answers the question, "What is it that I will try to prove in this piece?" Now, there are important points that you should take into account when composing your thesis statement.

1. **The thesis statement should be ideally written within the first paragraph; it is usually placed in the last sentence.** Because you are writing a 30-minute piece, you will not have the luxury of time to beat around the bush. Communicate the premise of your essay early on.

   Of course, there are essays where the thesis statement is declared in the last paragraph. Should you take this path, you have to ensure that you will hold the interest of your reader all throughout the piece or that your arguments are organised to fit this kind of structure. Nevertheless, this is only advisable if you are a skilled writer who has used this technique effectively in many practice attempts.

2. **The thesis statement should be clearly stated in the declarative format.** In some cases, an essay might pose a question; for example, "Should justice stay blind and impartial in all instances?" This is not exactly a thesis statement. The answer to this question <u>IS</u> the thesis

Medium-level Importance

statement. Hence you need to present your thesis in the declarative (e.g., "Justice cannot remain blind if the protection of the innocent is compromised.")

Again, because this is a (more or less) 30-minute writing task, you cannot waste time posing several questions because you will need to answer all of them. Otherwise, your essay will feel unresolved and indecisive. Remember that your task is to provide a definite standpoint - not just raise questions.

3. **A thesis statement should be a debatable claim to be proven using logical reasoning.** It should not be a statement about a generally accepted idea or fact. If you choose to make a generally accepted idea, your essay will fail to be a dialectic as you will likely struggle to present a sound antithesis. A failure to do so will naturally lead to a lower mark.

4. **A good thesis statement should cover a narrow scope of the topic.** If you embark on a very broad premise such as justice or parenting in general, you will either run out of time or overwhelm yourself with a plethora of evidences to offer in order to persuade your reader that your position is valid. The narrower the scope of your thesis, the more effective your argument will be. Again, the more general your thesis, the more difficult it will be to develop and respond to an antithesis.

Example of a factual statement: It is every parent's duty to guide his or her children onto the right path.

Example of a debatable and narrow thesis: Parents should refrain from becoming too close with their children if they want to develop emotionally resilient and responsible adults.

4.2.2 Writing an Interesting Introduction

"The beginning is the most important part of the work," according to Plato. How you write your essay's introduction is indeed critical. You either impress and arouse the markers' interest or you forewarn them that this is going to be a difficult read. This makes beginning the essay quite intimidating for some candidates. For others, generating the initial ideas itself is a struggle.

The good news is that you can remedy a scriptophobia of introductions by following an outline for writing your first paragraph. You can choose to adopt a logical introduction or a creative and catchy one.

- The Logical Introduction

Most discursive essays follow this type of introduction. Your main aim will be to set a logical connection between the main idea, which the comments express and the viewpoint you are taking.

It is also important to introduce the quote at this stage. This may seem redundant, however, it will give you an opportunity to demonstrate that you understand the idea being quoted. You will also be required to define the key term/s, especially if you are responding to them through a particular assumption. Do not be scared to address any parameters in the initial paragraph. For instance, you may decide to limit the discussion about justice to a particular area. By doing this, you are demonstrating to the marker that you have recognised the breadth of the theme, and you are choosing to thoroughly examine one aspect.

Sentence 1: state your interpretation of the comments' theme.

You can choose to write a summation of the comments' core idea or a paraphrase of one or two of the given comments. Alternatively, you can interlace a restatement of your selected quote.

Example:

A point of debate about the essence of justice is whether justice should remain unbiased or advocate for what is right.

Sentences 2 to 3: introduce the quote, and then define what the theme means in this context. Alternatively, expound the idea of the first sentence by citing the two sides of the argument.

A good formula to use for these two sentences would be to write something to this effect: *"Some say that . . . (quote or paraphrase one of the comments). Others say that . . . (quote or paraphrase another one of the comments)."*

Example 1:

Some say that justice cannot choose who it should favour. Others say that it should prompt one to always choose the right thing to do.

Example 2:

As Eleanor Roosevelt once said, "Justice cannot be for one side alone, but must be for both." On the other hand, proponents against this view will argue that justice cannot sacrifice the truth and the protection of the innocent.

Sentence 4: state which point of view you are taking. This is essentially your thesis statement.

Example:

Justice needs to be dispensed by going through the process of the legal system even if the end result does not suit everyone's ideal of justice.

Now let's put everything together and see if the introduction makes sense:

A point of debate about the essence of justice is whether justice should remain unbiased or advocate for what is right. Some say that justice cannot choose who it should favour. Others say that it should prompt one to always choose the right thing to do. Nevertheless, I believe that justice needs to be dispensed by going through the process of the legal system even if the end result does not suit everyone's ideal of justice.

- The Catchy Introduction

Another way to open your essay is by making it unique or striking. In an exam where thousands of papers are being marked, novelty and freshness of ideas can give your piece an edge. Uniqueness may also refer to presentation style. There are several creative devices to help you bait the markers' attention. We will discuss five of the most effective ones, namely: surprising facts or statistics, dramatic anecdotes, analogies or metaphors, thought-provoking questions, and powerful quotations.

However, please keep in mind that no matter which style you choose, you should not deviate from the the two main purposes of your introduction: to link the ideas between the comments and your own, and to articulate your point of view through a clear thesis statement.

1. Surprising fact or statistics

This approach requires adequate research and reading from various sources such as history, published research and the news.

Example 1:

In 16th century England, an otherwise loyal subject of Henry VIII uttered, "I like not the proceedings of this realm". For this, he was imprisoned.

Example 2:

On June 11, 1963, a Vietnamese Mahayana Buddhist monk named Thích Quang Duc burned himself to death in Saigon to protest the predominantly Catholic South Vietnamese government's persecution of Buddhists.

Example 3:

An article in The Economist in 2013 reported that ten people were killed in a fire in a factory used by famous foreign clothes retailers in the Bangladeshi capital. Bangladesh is the world's second largest supplier of clothes, yet three-fifths of its factories are far from being a risk-free work environment.

Example 4:

It takes 2400 litres of water to make one hamburger.

Example 5:

Every year, three times as much garbage is being dumped in oceans as the weight of fish caught.

Medium-level Importance

2. Dramatic anecdote

If you perceive yourself as someone with unique stories to tell, then this style might work for you. Basically, you begin your essay with an engaging narrative. It could be about a personal experience or an imagined scenario that depicts the essence of your response to the writing task.

If you do decide to adopt this introductory device, make sure to expose yourself to as many creative narrative styles. Practice regularly so that you develop the following key skills:

- Use of vivid, descriptive language
- Keeping the narrative concise yet entertaining

Creative introductions still follow the conventions of a standard introductory paragraph.

Example 1:

By the time I was five years old, I learnt all of The Beatles songs as my parents would always play their albums at home. One song particularly stood out to me - "Help!" In times of need during my five years in the world, I always had my friends to lend a helping hand, whether it be help to colour in my new art book or help to keep me from boredom when I played alone with my Barbie dolls. I could not imagine my life without help from my friends. After listening to John Lennon's song longing for friendship, I took it upon myself to respond. I proceeded to write an appealing letter to John letting him know that I would be delighted to be his friend - I would help him with his interest in music and he could voice my Ken dolls when we played my favourite game.

Example 2:

As I laid eyes on the tray of fresh fruits on our breakfast table this morning, I imagine a not-so-distant future when fruits take the form of morning shots instead. Natural food consumption would have become a luxury, reserved only for the privileged and moneyed. Farms and plantations would have all dried up and devoid of soil nutrients. Rain would have been only spoken in fairy tales. Earth would have been deprived of its once abundant blessings from Mother Nature; and so we have to create an artificial environment somewhere in space for plants to grow. Such are possibilities that I envision as I look at my morning fruits with global warming in the background.

3. Analogy, metaphor, simile

Analogies and metaphors are creative tools for thinking about a concept. They are usually effective in making a complicated idea or a very broad theme simpler to understand. You may also use this stylistic device if you want to give an old and tired concept a fresh treatment.

Basically, you have to choose a symbol or an equivalent situation that will embody the central point of your essay. Then you discuss it with an "as if" perspective. The trick is to use this symbol as a main reference throughout your paper. Refer back to it in the body as well as in the conclusion of your essay.

Reading creative literature frequently is a great way of honing the skillful use of analogies, metaphors and similes in an essay.

Example 1:

People attempt love like climbers attempt Mt. Everest. You struggle upward and end whenever and wherever you grow weary. If you do make it to the top to see the view, it is amazing; but most people will die trying. Love's dual nature . . .

Example 2:

A democratic government is like a boarding school. The lawmakers and public officials take the role of housemasters or mistresses in keeping the house and in overseeing its day-to-day running while you go on with your personal endeavours. You pay your taxes just like you would pay the boarding school fees; otherwise, the services will cease to fully operate. Citizens are also called to vote much like parents would be invited in a meeting for consultations on key issues. If you fail to show up in such a referendum, then you forfeit your opportunity to be heard. The balancing system in a democratic government is such that . . .

4. Thought-provoking question

Sometimes, an idea becomes all the more powerful when you inject some intrigue or controversy into it. This is what you intend to do when you pose a thought-provoking question at the start of your essay. But as already discussed, make sure to provide a clear answer to your own question during your main discussion. Remember that a question is only used here in order to emphasise a point. It is not up for the markers to answer or think about.

Examples:

Would you break the law to keep your country safe?

What will you say at your parents' funeral?

Is doing something wrong acceptable if no one is harmed anyway?

If money cannot buy happiness, can you be truly happy even without money?

5. Powerful quotation

"I quote others only in order to better express myself," DeMontaigne once said. A properly placed quotation can have a powerful effect on your Writing Task. If used improperly, you will have inadvertently confirmed that you misunderstood the statement provided.

You can choose to use a quotation to support your position or to provide the opposite point of view. But remember: the quotation must parallel the theme of the writing task, and a quote must be written word for word. Markers will not be impressed if you misquote John F. Kennedy or The Constitution. If you only forgot the name of someone who is not well-known, you can get away with saying something like: "It has been said that..."

Don't forget that even with creative introductions, responding to the comments' theme is still the central objective. You may also still need to expound on the idea brought forward by the surprising fact, the dramatic anecdote, the analogy, the thought-provoking question or the powerful quotation that you used. Basically, all of the ingredients of the logical introduction must remain while you add the extra creativity using the latter methods. Finally, the introductory paragraph must also be concluded by a strong thesis statement.

Here is an example of an introduction, which employs a dramatic anecdote in response to our previous quotes on parents:

My mother and I never really got along. I think it started when I was about five. My mother was suffering from palpitations and she kept telling me that my misbehaviours would aggravate her condition. Whenever she saw me, she noticed something wrong with what I wore or with what I was doing. She never told me she loved me, and she never hugged or kissed me - and to think that I was an only child. Surprisingly, the events following my mother's death would prove that parents do need to distance themselves from their children if it means teaching them to be emotionally resilient and to live responsibly.

The next sample introduction uses one of the interesting historical facts that we featured earlier. It is a response to the following comments:

* * * * *

Comment 1

A people which is able to say everything becomes able to do everything.
Napoleon Bonaparte

* * * * *

Comment 2

Freedom of Speech is ever the Symptom, as well as the Effect of a good Government.

Cato's Letters

* * * * *

Comment 3

To have a right to speak about something is not the same as to be in the right mind and position in saying it.

* * * * *

Comment 4

Free speech includes the right to not speak.

Jimmy Wales

* * * * *

Comment 5

Freedom of speech is a principal pillar of a free government.

Benjamin Franklin

In 16th century England, an otherwise loyal subject of Henry VIII uttered, "I like not the proceedings of this realm". For this, he was imprisoned. It is hard to imagine a time when people can be put to death for speaking their minds. Yet history has taught us that despite adverse consequences, free speech proves to be one of the most powerful indicators of democracy and a vehicle of positive change. Therefore, for a country like Australia to be considered a truly free society, it must amend its constitutional declaration of rights to include free speech or the freedom to express one's opinion publicly without fear of censorship or punishment.

If you want to practice formulating your own initial paragraph in response to a given set of comments, you can jump to the end of this chapter (WC 4.11) to find the Written Communication practice worksheet for writing an introduction.

4.2.3 Supporting Your Thesis

After you have established your view on the overall idea of the various comments, your next task is to provide reasons why you are choosing a particular stand (thesis). Each reason must be discussed in one paragraph and supported by an evidential example.

Consider the markers to be educated yet skeptically, neutral readers. They may not be hostile to your point of view. They may not also agree with all your assumptions and conclusions; but they certainly need to be convinced that your claim has logical bases. You must be able to show them that you can very well defend your views in an intelligent and systematic manner.

Hence the primary purpose of using examples is to strengthen your point. Do not enumerate an aimless list of events and all sorts of examples just to interpret a quote or define the theme. Every assertion you make in the essay must be substantiated, placed in concrete scenarios and logically argued in defence of your main thesis. **The key is in sifting the strongest and most relevant supporting examples.**

- Qualities of Effective Examples

The following is a list of factors to consider when choosing which examples to use in your supporting arguments.

1. Relevance

Everything you include in your essay should be about backing up the thesis statement. Stay on track. Always keep that thesis statement in mind when you discuss your examples. In addition, remember that whatever points you make in the body of your essay are meant to be synthesised in the concluding paragraph. If you discuss a number of unrelated ideas, this will result in a conclusion which is disorganised or characterised by redundant statements.

2. Balance

The evidence you present must include a full range of opinions about the issue. Your argument must not only be convincing but must also be well-rounded. Choose the strongest possible refutation to your thesis. However, do not say outright how the opposing views are wrong. Rather, examine one or two counterpoints and explain why you disagree with them. It could be because those views are biased or outdated. Be firm but maintain tact.

When done properly, including a counterargument gives your paper credibility. It means that you have thoroughly considered all possible assertions about the subject before arriving at an informed decision. It may seem counter-intuitive to detail arguments in refutation of your thesis; however, there exists sound reason to do so. Inclusion of an antithesis demonstrates critical thinking; it shows that you have thought about the weaknesses of your thesis, and it then allows you to defend your thesis in a new context. It is not enough to state your thesis and supporting examples, nor is it enough to simply discuss the "for" and "against" of your argument – the best essays will address one or more arguments in support of the thesis, an argument supporting the antithesis and then also address the shortcomings of this antithesis.

3. Accuracy

If necessary, cite data that are accurate and up-to-date. Include your sources. These will make your claims all the more real and valid.

● Different Types of Supporting Examples

There are several types of examples that you can use to build your argument, but it is important to understand how you can use them in conjunction with the three levels of appeals in reasoning:

Logos - is an appeal to the reader's mind and sense of reason because it employs factual and quantifiable evidence. Examples are drawn from research and wide reading hence they are predominantly objective. They become even more convincing when interpreted in the light of your thesis. This is the most common appeal used in argumentative essays.

The following are forms of factual evidence:

> **Real examples** drawn from history or current events

> **Statistics** such as those cited in surveys and case studies

> **Published research** from reputable journals and books

> **News Report**

Ethos - makes use of the writer's credibility or 'ethical appeal'. For example, if the theme speaks about environmental issues and you happen to have experience working in a climate change organisation, you might want to mention it in your essay. Just make sure that it is highly relevant in your discussion.

A usual form of evidence used in this level of appeal is an expert testimony:

> **Expert testimony** or opinion coming from a reputable source in a specialised field

In this case, the quality of evidence is just as important as the credibility of the source. Would you believe information cited in The Economist rather than from a student newsletter?

Ethos can also be achieved through the use of an authoritative tone, as well as sophisticated language.

Pathos - appeals to the reader's emotions and imagination. One of the most effective means to convey pathos is through a narrative in which the reader can sympathise and even identify with the writer's point of view. It should be evident by now that an argument can take the form of a narrative or a reflective essay if your main objective is to prove a point. Pathos, when appropriately used in conjunction with ethos, can be quite powerful.

> **Narrative** drawn from first-hand experience

Take note that a personal example is only material in an argumentative piece if it is able to illustrate the main assertion that you want to make. Moreover, this type of justification would be ideal to use when more objective and more logical sources of evidence are not available. In this instance, the validity of an argument cannot be easily questioned because it is based on a "lived experience". Further, a personal narrative must be emotionally, psychologically or spiritually poignant.

- Forming Opinions

The importance of reading a wide range of topics cannot be stressed enough. Your choice of reading materials should include opinion articles from reputable newspapers and magazines, books on political theories and even philosophical essays. However, do not just take note of possible supporting examples, which you can get from these sources. Aside from reading for the purpose of exposing yourself to different issues and concepts, you also need to develop the habit of forming your own judgement based on what the writers are saying. This second purpose is the essence of the Written Communication writing tasks.

Some successful candidates in the past reveal that they engage in journal writing as part of their Written Communication preparation. If you have the time to emulate this strategy, you can keep a notebook where you can write out your thoughts about certain events, debates, and other writer's opinions on current issues. Do you agree with them? Why or why not? What do these issues mean to you? How do these issues affect you or members in your community?

4.2.4 Organisation and Structure

Keeping a logical organisation of your thoughts is another important element in building an argument. It allows the marker to have a clear vision of your reasoning process. Moreover, an orderly, sound explanation of each argued point adds weight to your claims.

It is also essential to keep in mind that Written Communication is a timed writing test. Following a prepared format for your writing tasks will save you time in planning what to do. Instead, you can just focus on developing quality content and still maintain coherence throughout the piece. We will discuss this further in the next sections.

Of course, you have to practice using an essay template as many times as you can prior to the actual sitting. The earlier you practice using a certain template, the better chance for you to get so used to writing in an organised manner such that you would become confident enough to experiment injecting your own style.

Nevertheless, do not forget that structure precedes style. A reader will be less likely to appreciate a stylish but disorganised essay. One idea must flow smoothly to the next. You have to be able to indicate properly if you are about to shift your line of argument or extend it with a detailed discussion.

There are "transitional cues" that you can use depending on your purpose in the different paragraphs. The following usually apply, although they are not limited to the first paragraph and its supporting paragraphs:

To place what you just said in a particular context: in this connection, in relation to, in this perspective

To give an example or an illustration: for example, for instance, in this case, to illustrate, as an illustration, take the case of, to take another example, namely, that is, as shown by, as illustrated by, as expressed by

To offer a similar point: similarly, in other words, likewise, in a similar manner, like, in the same way

The following are commonly found in the paragraph that offers a counterargument:

To show contrast: however, nevertheless, rather, whereas, on the other hand, on the contrary, but, yet, although, conversely, meanwhile, in contrast, otherwise, one may object that . . .

To compare: by comparison, compared to, balanced against, vis a vis, alternatively

The next transitional cues are mostly used towards the concluding paragraphs:

To refer back to an earlier point: as I have said, in brief, as I have noted, as indicated earlier, as has been noted

To express a resolution: granted, naturally, of course, in any case

To prove your point: for the same reason, obviously, evidently, indeed, in fact

To show cause and effect: as a result, consequently, hence, therefore, due to, for this reason

To conclude: on the whole, to sum up, to conclude, in conclusion, as I have shown, as I have said

The next list of transitional cues are used in any part of an essay as deemed necessary:

To add something: further, furthermore, equally important, moreover, in addition, not only . . . but also

To introduce a new idea: furthermore, moreover, in addition

To emphasise an idea: indeed, definitely, extremely, undeniably, absolutely, obviously, surprisingly, without a doubt, certainly

The last paragraph is your last shot at convincing the markers that your essay deserves a high score. Summarise the major points discussed in the preceding paragraphs so that your ideas follow a logical conclusion. Never introduce any new ideas or another example. Instead, address any questions posed in the essay. Then restate your thesis using different words and in the light of the various arguments presented.

The next two sections will now focus on the format of the two writing tasks (A and B).

4.2.5 Focussing on Task A

Let "A" be Argumentative!

In the current GAMSAT, there is no strict imposition coming from ACER that candidates should adhere to a certain style. However, the argumentative (thesis – antithesis – resolution) or discursive (pro – con – resolution) formats prove to be the most effective in dealing with socio-cultural topics.

Moreover, as a candidate seeking admission to a medical education (a science-based degree!), you should be able to display an ability to be objective in weighing the pros and cons of various arguments.

An argumentative essay has three tasks. These tasks are summarised below:

Gold Standard Structure for Writing Test A

1. **Thesis:** the first paragraph should provide an explanation or an interpretation of the theme. You may also include one or two quotations that you have chosen, followed by an expression of your position on the point of issue. The second paragraph (and sometimes a 3rd) provides an example, real or hypothetical, that supports your thesis.

2. **Antithesis:** the next paragraph or paragraphs evaluate opposing views to the one presented in the Thesis.

3. **Synthesis:** the final paragraph concludes with a way for the conflict between the viewpoint expressed in the Thesis and the one presented in the Antithesis to be reconciled.

These three tasks should keep you quite busy for approximately 30 minutes that you have to write the essay. The tasks, however, once you are familiar with them, will help you by structuring your essay automatically.

Alternatively, you can follow a detailed outline, which can serve as either a Writing Task A template or a checklist to make sure that the essay meets all the requirements. In any case, having a framework of presentation allows you to actually think of the substance as the form has already been prepared.

Gold Standard Detailed Structure (Test A)

Paragraph 1: Open with a thesis statement.

a. Paraphrase the comment you are responding to. You can state it as a regular statement or you may use a creative device.

b. Explain what the comment means to you in light of the overall theme.

c. State your agreement or disagreement with this main idea. This is your expression of the thesis statement.

Paragraph 2: Provide support for your thesis.

a. Give the reason why you agree or disagree with the comments.

b. Explain what your argument is and provide an example or examples to support them.

c. Explain how the examples relate to the arguments.

Paragraph 3: Discuss an antithesis to your main idea.

a. Cite the strongest argument against your main idea.

b. Discuss it so that you can show the marker that you are capable of 'reasoning' through objections and observations that may put your arguments in jeopardy.

c. Provide an illustration of the counterargument.

Paragraph 4: Explain why you stay firm with your thesis.

a. Demolish the antithesis by showing its weaknesses against your arguments in support of the thesis.

b. Alternatively, you can cite situations in which your thesis best applies and in which instances the antithesis can be appreciated.

Paragraph 5: Conclude your essay.

a. Tie up all the ideas and present it for the consideration of the reader.

b. You may propose a plan of action or a course of action so that the reader can act upon your ideas.

c. You can also invite the reader to agree with you.

You may also want to use Written Communication Practice Worksheet III (Task A Template) found in WC 4.11 as a guide every time you practice writing your Task A responses.

Why not the expository format?

The Written Communication section assesses your thinking process in forming your views on the given themes. An expository essay simply explains an idea, a theme or an issue. Explanations may show your vast knowledge on a subject but not necessarily your ability to form judgments.

An argumentative or discursive essay, on the other hand, involves the process of establishing a claim (your thesis statement) and then proving it with the use of logical reasoning, examples, and research.

The following are two sample responses to the quotations on justice. The sample responses were both written by students within the prescribed time limit. Just as an additional exercise, after reading the instructions and quotations, you should try completing an essay in 30 minutes prior to reviewing the two sample responses.

Note: There does not exist one format that everyone should use. We are presenting formats that would optimise the score of most candidates.

Confidence and skill level may lead you to apply your own approach with or without creativity. The key is to practice your chosen approach and improve with time.

Writing Task A

Read the following statements and write a response to any one or more of the ideas presented.

Your essay will be evaluated on the value of your thoughts on the theme, logical organisation of content and effective articulation of your key points.

* * * * *

Comment 1

Justice is justly represented blind, because she sees no difference in the parties concerned.

William Penn

* * * * *

Comment 2

Justice cannot be for one side alone, but must be for both.

Eleanor Roosevelt

* * * * *

Comment 3

It is better that ten guilty persons escape than one innocent suffer.

William Blackstone

* * * * *

Comment 4

It is more important that innocence be protected than it is that guilt be punished, for guilt and crimes are so frequent in this world that they cannot all be punished.

John Adams

* * * * *

Comment 5

Justice consists not in being neutral between right and wrong, but in finding out the right and upholding it, wherever found, against the wrong.

Theodore Roosevelt

Sample Response 1 (Discursive Essay)

The Net of Justice: Selective or Unselective?

Even if guilty men walk free, justice is done provided the innocent avoid punitive measures. This was the notion expressed by judge and author of the Commentaries on the Laws of England William Blackstone when he declared, "It is better that ten guilty persons escape than one innocent suffer." From this perspective one can define justice to be served only when the guilty are punished, and the innocent unaffected. While some proponents of Blackstone's view argue that this is the only way justice can be achieved, there are those who advocate that justice necessitates castigating some of the innocent. The following dialectic will urge that justice can only be achieved if the innocent remain unscathed in the pursuit of justice.

When the guilty and innocent fail to be differentiated, injustice occurs. It is reasonable to hold this view because the innocent are necessarily punished for crimes that they have not committed. If society does not discriminate between the guilty and the innocent, it either grants freedom to all or freedom to none, and it is clear that both situations fail to amount to justice. For example, the sexual abuse scandals in the Catholic Church over the last few decades have been cause for great communal debate. Initially the heinous crimes against children had been ignored by senior figures from within the church. At this point, justice was not affected upon the individual perpetrators, and this has primed the contemporary state. Today, it has become very difficult to prosecute the perpetrators of sexual abuse due to the amount of time that has passed. The result of this injustice and constant revelation of new scandal from the past has led to an undercurrent of hatred and anger for the Catholic Church that is perhaps unwarranted when one considers that only very few of their congregation actually committed crimes. This notion is also evident in the newly enacted laws restricting the associative activities of motorcycle clubs in Queensland. Though members may not be criminals themselves, they are treated as such due to their association with gangs labelled 'outlaws'. In these instances, one can see that the failure to sequester the guilty and the innocent can lead to great injustice as either the guilty are free, or the innocent are punished.

Conversely, there exists merit for countervailing arguments, especially given the complexity of the subject that is justice. Some argue that in some instances it is necessary to prosecute both the guilty and the innocent in pursuit of justice. This notion might be exemplified in areas such as sport where athletes are forced to endure mandatory drug testing at any hour of the day or night. In this situation, all are considered guilty before they have even laid step onto their respective sporting arenas. Though this view is understandable, the example of drugs in sport is more an anomaly than a rule, and the damages to the innocent are rather insignificant when the higher purpose is considered. The invalidity of this greater argument becomes apparent when one applies this rule to subjects such as the mandatory detention of asylum seekers. All asylum seekers whether legitimate or fraudulent are processed through the same means: off shore, within a dangerous penitentiary and with a long wait. Asylum seekers legitimately seeking refuge from the flames and bullets of their homelands find no sanctuary due to these inappropriate processes and the plight of those afflicted by this unjust process exemplifies the shortcoming inherent in the notion that it is acceptable to punish the innocent in the pursuit of the guilty.

Thus, justice can only be achieved when the guilty are differentiated and prosecuted. When this fails to occur, so does justice as exhibited by the current plight of the Catholic Church and Queensland motorcycle clubs. Though there are anomalous instances where it may be acceptable to net the innocent with the guilty, this rule usually applies to instances where the imposition is insignificant and is not applicable across greater society. Therefore, it is difficult to find difference with Blackstone's view.

Sample Response 2 (Persuasive Essay)

The Justice System

Justice depends upon fallible humans applying imperfect laws, thus, justice is imperfect. But without the justice system, without the laws and the rules, society will break down and anarchy will reign.

We call it a "system" because dispensing justice involves several steps, several procedures and several people. There are legislators who make laws that define what behaviours are deemed to be criminal acts. There are police officers who enforce these criminal laws and apprehend persons thought to be violating the law. Then there are prosecutors who weigh the availability of evidence as well as the admissibility of the evidence gathered by the police. The prosecutors decide if there is enough evidence to obtain a conviction and file indictments based on the evidence gathered. The accused are afforded the right to retain their own lawyer so that they can put up a defence. The accused are given their day in court to face their accusers. The judge decides what pieces of evidence can be considered by the court or by the jury. The jury decides if the evidence presented gives them a moral certainty that a crime was indeed committed by the person accused of it.

Justice is not simple. There are concepts such as "innocent until proven guilty" and the "right against self-incrimination" that ensure that each accused person is afforded due process of law before he is found guilty. Ultimately, justice is practical: is there enough evidence to prove that a crime has been committed and that the accused committed the crime? This is all that should matter.

Of course, it is also true that when the accused is poor, he has not the resources to hire a lawyer of his choice. He usually is assigned a lawyer by the court. Because he is poor, he does not have money to ensure that he obtains all the evidence and all the expert testimony necessary to present a credible defence. When the accused is rich, he has all the resources to hire the best lawyers, and he has the money to challenge every piece of evidence presented by the prosecution.

Justice under the law is not true justice. It is judicial justice. It is not unheard of that a person who truly committed a crime has been acquitted because there was no sufficient evidence to convict him beyond reasonable doubt. It is not unheard of either that a person who has not committed a crime has been found guilty of having committed one. Justice often boils down to the impression made on the jury. It is the perception of the jury that matters whether or not a person will be found guilty or not guilty.

A jury consists of ordinary men and women who swear to hear evidence and evaluate it according to set rules and to determine if the evidence presented is enough to find the accused guilty. If any member of the jury has any mental reservation at all, then there can be no conviction. This is the rule of reasonable doubt. If any member of the jury has any doubt as to the probable guilt of the accused, then, the accused will have to be acquitted.

Justice is lofty not in the result but in the effort with which we ensure that it is carried out. Yes, occasionally, a guilty man may be acquitted and yes, an innocent man may be convicted. This does not mean that there is no justice. Justice cannot always be done, but justice must be served by going through the process of the justice system even if the end result does not suit everybody's sense of justice.

4.2.6 Focussing on Task B

Let "B" be Bersonal? OK, it does not exactly spell "personal" but it's close enough! The important point is to understand that you may attempt a different approach in the second writing task. But then again, nothing stops you from utilising the argumentative style in Task B.

Why so different?

Consider some of the criticisms aimed at young doctors: impressive "book knowledge" and technical ability but lacking skills in listening, communicating and empathising. Is it a fact that younger people are less empathetic because of a lack of experience? Can interpersonal skills - including empathy - be the focus of a section of a standardised exam? How does one evaluate empathy?

Ideas and imagination

They need to know whether you can imagine someone else's perspective. This does not mean that you need to write a creative story using the imagination of Isaac Asimov! It simply means that you have to be able to visualise and explain how other people may be feeling and experiencing life; thus the personal-interpersonal and social theme.

Introspection and Reasoning

The logical presentation of your views on the theme (i.e. your reasoning process) will still be part of the marking criteria in Task B. You can also demonstrate empathy using the discursive format. On the other hand, you may find that using pathos through personal reflection would be more effective in supporting your thesis.

A personal reflection is a narrative about a remarkable event in your life. It can be your own experience or one that involved a close friend or a family member. It must be recounted with enough details in order to help the readers understand where your perspectives are coming from. However, it should neither read like a confession nor a diary. Rather, it should serve as an example from which you can extract life-lessons that are germane to the theme.

Unlike a pure narrative or a creative non-fiction, you have to be explicit in your realisations, perceptions, and opinions. This personal example is your proof, taken from first-hand experience, to validate a point that you are trying to make. In addition, it should highlight a shift in perspectives or a fresh insight into a prevalent interpersonal-social problem such as bullying, domestic violence, discrimination and the likes.

Extending your personal realisations to a social issue exhibits another aspect of reasoning ability: the ability to be mentally resilient. When you can learn from an experience, take a personal truth and apply it to a novel situation, you are showing that you can continue to educate yourself outside formal teaching, adapt ideas and make them work under different circumstances.

The Personal and Social Relevance

When discussing the social issue part in your essay, it might help to imagine as if you are talking to a patient or a relative of a patient who is in a challenging condition. The person may be feeling frustrated, discriminated, or starting to lose self-esteem because of a debilitating disease. In this case, you would like to share your story as a possible source of inspiration.

The conversation can go something like "I (or my friend) once was. . . But I came to realise that . . . so then I decided to . . . and now I feel that (state a possible solution based on your personal triumph). . ." Of course this is just one strategy. An alternative would be to pick a quote from the given comments that easily pose a personal-social significance. This way, both themes can be interwoven in a single thread of discussion.

The organisation of the Task B essay can be summarised as follows:

Gold Standard Structure for Writing Test B

1. **Introduction:** the first paragraph should acquaint the reader with the topic. In addition, it should give the markers a glimpse of what to expect from the body of your text, which you can do by clearly stating your specific assertion and point of view. Make sure your introduction is written in an active tone, with strong verbs and powerful statements.

2. **The body:** the second paragraph (and sometimes a 3rd and/or 4th) should focus on one main idea that supports your assertions in the Introduction. Dissect that main idea into three distinct parts: the main assertion, a specific supporting example or examples, and a summary (each could be one paragraph depending on how much you can write effectively in the limited time).

3. **Conclusion:** the last paragraph summarises the main point(s), reasserts your view and ends the essay with impact. This will be the last thing markers will get from your essay, so make sure it ties everything together succinctly as well as creates a lasting impression in their mind.

High-level Importance

High-level Importance

Remember to write your Task B with feeling.

The following is a more detailed outline in writing a personal reflection:

Gold Standard Detailed Structure (Test B)

Paragraph 1: Begin with a thesis statement.

a. Paraphrase the comments. Explain what they mean to you in light of the overall theme.

b. State whether you agree or disagree with the main idea in the comments and why.

c. Briefly discuss one argument that supports your stance. This is the transitional sentence for you to introduce your narrative. Your personal experience of an event or a condition will be your main argument.

Paragraph 2: Begin the narrative.

a. This is your personal illustration thus it must be written in your own point of view (avoid the third person).

b. It must be a story of something that happened to you or to someone very close to you and which you experienced vicarious pain or joy, stress, discomfort or fear.

c. You must choose an event that is rich with emotion and one that is pivotal in your life.

Note: Sometimes, the narrative can take several paragraphs.

Paragraph 3: Reflect upon the narrative you just described.

a. You must say what you learned from the narrative or experience.

b. Describe how you felt, how you thought and what made you change your mind or your perspective.

c. There must be a 'before-and-after' description of your state of mind and state of heart.

Paragraph 4: Apply the reflection or life-lesson you learned.

a. Find a problem that is relevant to the problem you described in your narrative.

b. The problem must be something that affects a large segment of society.

c. Your life-lesson can be an insight you can share with those people who may be similarly situated; it could be a source of inspiration or a challenge for them.

Written Communication Practice Worksheet IV found in WC 4.11 corresponds to a Task B Template. You can use it as a guide when attempting your Task B essays. We have placed two sample responses to the quotations on parenting or parents' love. They were both written within the prescribed time limit. Consider attempting the 30-minute essay before assessing the sample responses.

Writing Task B

Read the following statements and write a response to any one or more of the ideas presented.

Your essay will be evaluated on the value of your thoughts on the theme, logical organisation of content and effective articulation of your key points.

* * * * *

Comment 1

Parents are always more ambitious for their children than they are for themselves.

* * * * *

Comment 2

We never know the love of a parent till we become parents ourselves.

Henry Ward Beecher

* * * * *

Comment 3

Parents can only give good advice or put them on the right paths, but the final forming of a person's character lies in their own hands.

Anne Frank

* * * * *

Comment 4

Some mothers are kissing mothers and some are scolding mothers, but it is love just the same, and most mothers kiss and scold together.

Pearl S. Buck

* * * * *

Comment 5

A father's goodness is higher than the mountain, a mother's goodness deeper than the sea.

Japanese Proverb

Sample Response 1 (Reflective Essay)

Every time I saw my father, I saw disappointment in his eyes. And why should he not be disappointed? He spent for my education through grade school, high school, university and post graduate studies in law. I was a lawyer and I left my law practice to tend to my sick son. It was once said that "parents are always more ambitious for their children than they are for themselves." However, I believe that the way I live my life, raise my own family and define success is still up to me.

My son developed jaundice on the second day of his life because there was bile sludge in his bile duct. He needed surgery and after the successful surgery, he needed follow-up. I was at the peak of my career, but I made the difficult decision to concentrate on nursing my son back to health instead of going to court everyday and leaving my sick son in the care of strangers.

I was a full-time and hands-on kind of mother. I breastfed the baby, changed him, cleaned him, played with him and rocked him to sleep. I read to him, sang to him and talked to him. We were inseparable. I was with him to every doctor's appointment. I held him and comforted him through every inoculation and every blood test. This was militant mother's love – the kind that is untiring in promoting and ensuring the health and well-being of her child.

I did this 24/7. I wanted to go back to work when he was about a year old but I found myself pregnant with my second child. I thought to myself that it was unfair to mother my son militantly and then leave my daughter to be raised by strangers. I did it all over again. Instead of having one child to care for, I had two. I did it every day for years that it became second nature to think of my children first before thinking of myself.

My own mother told me that I was cruising for a major disappointment because I was pouring myself into my children. She said that if I poured my entire being into my children, imprinting into them my very person, I would exhaust myself and then there would be no strength left for me. My mother said that someday, these children I had loved so intensely will grow up and leave and then, where would I be? I'd be left empty with no sense of achievement that I can proudly share with my own family.

I did not say a word when my mother said that. I did not argue with her. It made me understand her – that is why my mother was always stand-offish. All the while I was growing up, I felt that she was keeping something back from me, pulling from me each time we could be close. I thought she didn't really like me. Now I know. She loved me, but she just couldn't pour herself into me because she was afraid I would leave her one day. The result was that I had gotten accustomed to turn to myself for comfort and affection because I did not get sufficient comfort, attention or affection from my mother. I grew up without her, and I learned to fend for myself without her. Now that she is old, she reaches out to me, she wants us to hang out but there is just no love or affection between us - there is just nothing there on which to build a meaningful relationship upon.

My mother may be right – now that my kids are grown up, they go to school on their own, they go out with friends more often, and I'm left on my own again. I feel like my world is shaking – I am beginning to feel orphaned and naked. My children were like leaves on my tree and flowers on my bush. When they leave, I would be purposeless and meaningless. My life would be without prettiness because I think that my children made my life pretty. I like having them around, and I think they like having me around, too. They tell me things they wouldn't tell others. They ask me things they do not dare ask others. When they leave my nest, my nest will be empty.

So what should I do then? I've already done it – I got myself a dog. Dogs cannot take the place of my children, but they do fill the space and the hours when my kids are away. The dogs are there so that I'd have something to keep me occupied while I wait for my kids to come home. They really can't stay away too long – they are sure they will get love and attention here from me. I realise that I didn't take care of my children because they were mine and I was their mother. I took care of my children because that is who I am – I am a person who derives pleasure and meaning from taking care of others. In taking care of them, I was effectively actualising myself.

Mothering was what I was meant to do, this was what I was meant to be – I am a mother. And a mother's job is to raise kids so strong that they can survive without her. My mother and I just went about raising our kids in different ways: I would like to think that we both raised kids so strong they can survive without us. The only difference is, my kids would rather not survive without me. I have made their lives pretty just as they made mine pretty. That is the only difference.

High-level Importance

Sample Response 2 (Discursive Essay)

Parenting As a Social Responsibility

Would you starve your own daughter until she masters a very difficult lesson? This is what American lawyer, book author, and Yale Law School professor Amy Chua almost did to her younger daughter. In her book **Battle Hymn of the Tiger Mother**, Amy Chua confesses having a highly authoritarian parenting style. In one extreme situation, she did not allow her daughter, Lulu, to get up - not even for water or for bathroom breaks - until Lulu perfected playing a difficult piano piece. Professor Chua justifies her methods, claiming it is all about believing in your child more than they believe in themselves and making them realise their own potentials.

On the other hand, we've also heard of parents adopting a more positive and affectionate child-rearing style and advocates the same aspirations that Professor Chua hopes to achieve. Certainly, parents often have to use "carrot and stick" in order to instill discipline and values in a child. In any case, they are driven by one common reason: they love their children hence they will do whatever it takes to turn them into better and successful individuals. However, I do not agree that parenting should just be about developing your child's full potential and securing his or her bright future. Parenting should also be about raising children who will eventually become positive contributions to society.

Open communication and reasoning - explaining to a child the reasons why he or she is being pushed to the limits and at times punished - are quite important in developing individuals who are not merely focussed on self-improvement but also on the welfare and the rights of others. An example of this inductive approach is when a child - let's name him Andy - is found taking his classmate Ben's lunch without permission and worse, he does not own up to the misdemeanour. As his punishment, Andy is not allowed to watch TV and play video games for a month. But his parents also discuss crucial questions with him ranging from "How could have Ben possibly felt when he didn't have anything to eat during lunch?" to "How would your classmates and teachers feel now that they have someone in class whom they can no longer trust?"

Of course, the next time Andy feels like committing a similar misconduct, he would not only remember the punishment but also the uncomfortable thoughts and feelings attributed to the act: "I'd feel bad if someone did that to me. . . I don't want to lose their trust again. . . Our family does not take what's not ours." Hence Andy would discourage himself from misbehaving again. The benefits of inductive discipline for developing pro-social behaviour is further supported by a study conducted by Krevans and Gibbs in 1996. Their case study shows that parents who explain to their children the reasons and consequences of bad behaviour tend to develop empathy early in a child. These children also exhibit more self-control, moral reasoning, and consideration of how others feel.

The same approach can be employed when encouraging a child to excel in a skill. Instead of using pressure and threats, the parent draws from positive reinforcement and reasoning: “If you practiced real hard today, you’ll be able to perfect your piano piece very shortly. We’ll have time to go to the beach this weekend, and you’ll still be all set for a superb performance next week! Everyone’s happy.” Or better yet, a socially responsible parent would be able to reinforce his or her teenager’s decision to take up a health-related course that will help treat a disabled sibling and others with the same affliction.

Nonetheless, some child psychologists believe that moral reasoning may not always work with children who either have stronger and fearless temperament or too weak and fearful. Children who take on an adventurous outlook on life will take risks in repeating their offences. In this case, discipline may take more than explanations and simple punishment. Even emotional support may have to be in the form of firm rules and ultimatums. This is probably what drove Amy Chua to resort to extreme measures with her daughter, Lulu, who she described as a “real fireball”.

Another danger of moralising and reasoning especially to a young child is when an act of punishment is not properly processed. Parents are by no means developmental experts and may use words and situations that are not age-appropriate. For example, a five-year-old girl caught taking her friend’s favourite toy without permission may be made to think of the consequences of stealing. The concept of stealing may not even be fully clear at this age. This could result to confusion and unwarranted guilt on the part of the child.

Despite these contrary opinions on inductive parenting, open communication remains an effective tool in shaping socially and morally responsible children - and families. Even Amy Chua admits that her need to reach out to her daughter Lulu, who was rebelling at the time, served as the impetus to her (in)famous book. Showing the manuscript of her book to her husband and her daughters was cathartic to their family and saved their relationships. In the same manner, a parent who constantly talks and reasons with his or her child would know the most appropriate types of punishment and motivation to carry out. Hence, the argument against over-moralising would be more of a few exceptions than the rule.

In the end, it all boils down to a parent’s sense of purpose. If one is to merely mould a self-actualised individual and overlook the social responsibility that comes with raising a child, then any parenting method would do as long as the results are achieved. On the other hand, if one is to inculcate moral and social sensibility in a child, then open communication and moral reasoning should be a significant component of a family. The hope is that, as a child grows to adulthood, and as the presence of an authority figure correspondingly fades, he or she will develop a sense of internal moral compass to reason his or her way through life's dilemmas rather than be on the lookout for any external promise of reward or threat of punishment.

Notes on Writing Task B Sample Response #2

The second essay reflects upon a personal issue that the writer feels strongly about. Using the third person (instead of the first person point of view) does not diminish the strong personal conviction of the writer that underlies each and every single idea expressed. While the essay is about child rearing, it cannot be overlooked that the author is actually formulating an opinion on child discipline based upon strongly-held personal beliefs which the author then measures up against the standards of psychological theories. It is implied that the author is actually reacting to the extreme form of child rearing that s/he not only heard about or read about, the author may actually be reacting to the insensitive and inattentive parenting that he or she witnesses all around.

The essay also works (despite its argumentative stance) because it highlights the social responsibility of parenting. That is to say, the author's ideas on how children should be raised is extrapolated to the way we, as a society, is equipping the next generation to learn discernment and circumspection in choosing how we behave and how we make decisions. This is (obliquely) a commentary on a social issue that confronts us: undisciplined children who grow up to be lawless adults; the lack of standards of behaviour that allow our children to conclude that they can do whatever they wish without thought of consequences.

Over all, this essay works because it is an educated opinion that is logically presented and organised. The control of language is superb even if there are a few grammatical errors. It has a clear message, and it conveys that message quite forcefully. It paints a good picture for the marker to take away after reading the essay. It shows a picture of us as a society, and it lays the accountability for our failure, as parents, to ensure reason and reasonableness in our children. The examples may not be gleaned from the writer's actual life experiences for it to be potent but because the examples are so commonplace, we see it every day; and therefore, readers can relate to the examples.

4.2.7 Timing

Timing skills should be developed during the early stages of your Written Communication preparation. Be careful not to get too engrossed in developing your great ideas that you might neglect containing those thoughts within a limited time. You need to be able to get used to efficiently typing two well-organised essays on two different themes within 65 minutes.

Getting used to writing within the time limit will teach you to include only the most pertinent and strongest arguments in your essays. Note that you are in control as to how to allocate the time. Of the full 65 minutes to complete the two writing tasks, you might choose to spend 20 minutes on Task A and then 45 minutes on Task B. You must use your judgement, based on experience gained through practice, to optimise your GAMSAT score.

Indeed, some students can generate ideas easier on issues involving socio-cultural concerns and can thus finish Task A in less than 30 minutes. Others can be quite persuasive using a narrative. Still, others are more efficient discussing a well-balanced presentation of pros and cons. You will learn which essay format or style will be the easiest for you to control if you have practiced writing in a timed setting way beforehand.

Efficient Typing

Remember that GAMSAT is no longer a paper-based exam. As a result of the 2020 global pandemic, GAMSAT was converted to a digital exam accessible as home proctored (WC) and held at test centres with computers. Students who have not been practicing enough are sometimes surprised at their low typing efficiency (relatively slow speed with an abnormally high rate of errors). Add lack of real-exam experience, with annoying environmental sounds, and the result could be a reduction in your typing efficiency (side note: some test centres permit earplugs).

If you are used to writing by hand, typing essays might be challenging and can even affect your thinking process. Practice! If you do not have confidence in your typing skills, watch some videos on YouTube or use an interactive app to improve your speed and reduce the typographical errors. Just like any skill, timed essay-writing can be done in small stages. The trick is to do it consistently.

As of the time of this book's publication, there is no copy/paste function for the real exam.

When you begin practicing writing essays, do not worry about whether or not you'll be able to come up with an excellent piece. Just get yourself used to thinking spontaneously and then wrapping up your main points within the limited time. To help keep your thoughts organised, use the practice worksheets found in the last section of this chapter.

Next, examine your writing carefully and identify your weaknesses. Analyse what could be the causes. Is it a lack of exposure to current news? Could it be because you are uncomfortable with the format? Perhaps, you have problems arranging your ideas. It might also help to have someone you know or respect examine your writing effort.

Once you know what your weaknesses are, you can address them one at a time. Continue to practice writing essays on a regular basis but aim to improve at least one aspect for every attempt.

Finally, if you still have ample time for preparation, practice, practice, and practice to a point when you can almost tell how many minutes have elapsed as you get to Paragraph 1, to Paragraph 2, and so forth. Most successful candidates arrive to sit the test having completed 20-40 essays. While this may sound significant, there is much to be gained by writing and rewriting up to fifty essays. By doing so, you will arrive with a much greater body of knowledge and a strong faith in your structures.

4.2.8 The Gold Standard Five-minute, Five-step Plan

Another important component of your Written Communication strategy, which is quite related to timing, is pre-planning. We know that while it is possible to write a structured, complete essay in 30 minutes, this requires practice for most students. This is because normally, an essay would be written over a considerable period of time. You would think about your essay, plan what you would write, actually write, correct and polish your essay, and perhaps rewrite sections.

However, a timed essay is not normal. It is a situation where your thoughts have to be ordered, structured and organised straight out of your head! You have to plan what you will write quickly and efficiently. This is what the Gold Standard Five-minute, Five-step Plan is all about. The objective is for you to take 5 minutes to prepare and 5 steps to finish the essay.

Step 1: Read the instructions and the stimulus material.

This may seem obvious, but you would be surprised by the number of students who misread or misinterpret what is expected of them. Carefully read the quotations presented for both Writing Task A and Writing Task B.

As "scratch paper," you will be using either two A4 sheets of paper or an erasable whiteboard. Consider keeping something similar on your desk to jot down notes. Mentally or actually take notes related to the keywords from the quotations. Then look at the relationships of each idea in the different comments. Actively ask yourself the following questions: How does this particular idea relate to the other ideas? Do they contradict or support each other? If they contradict each other, what is the debatable issue that must be addressed? If they all agree with each other, what is the unifying theme that ties them all together? Earlier, we mentioned having completed as many essays as possible. By doing so, you will increase your chances of being able to use material from one of your practice essays.

Consider the following quotations and create an essay in response to one or more of them.

Example of a quotation that could be chosen from stimulus material in Writing Task A:

The government is best that governs least.

Henry David Thoreau

Now, in your mind, you should be thinking of writing a comprehensive essay in which you accomplish the following objectives. Explain what you think the statement means. Describe a specific example in which the government's powers should be increased. Discuss the basis for increasing or decreasing the government's powers. The preceding outlines the structure of the 'classic' argumentative essay (WC 4.2.5).

Step 2: Prewrite your Thesis (Task 1), Antithesis (Task 2) and Synthesis (Task 3).

Once the actual testing time starts, you should jot down notes on your scratch paper. Make your notes clear. As a habit, write the letter A and circle it for Task A, and write the letter B and circle it for Task B. Separate your work with a dividing line or by using different pages. As of the time of publication, the rule is that you may use two A4 sheets of paper or a laminated whiteboard. That is ample space to express ideas, but it is safer to develop good habits.

Generating ideas at this early stage will have the greatest impact on your final score.

Task 1: Usually, you will have to explain a statement which will not be simply factual or self-evident. For example, the statement, "The government is best which governs least," has to be explained and terms have to be defined. Make notes as the information comes to mind:

Ex.: Government: *-federal, state, provincial, municipal*
-authority, power; a ruling body

Governs: - *rules, delegates, guides*
-creates laws
-exerts control, authority

When it comes time to write (Step 4), you will formulate a statement which clearly addresses Task 1: "Explain what you think the statement means." You should choose one clear definition from amongst the possibilities. You may also want to use an example to further illustrate the point of view you are presenting:

The ideal ruling body would strive to maintain, at a minimum, its exertion of authority over the population. Clearly, a government representing the people should not have the right to indiscriminately curb the freedom of an individual. The consequence would be a contra-

diction of democratic principles. Thus a government should avoid extending its powers; rather, government should use its authority prudently.

There are many different interpretations and examples which can be used to explain what the statement means. One possibility is to suggest that 'big' government produces excessive 'red tape' or bureaucracy which eventually may lead to higher taxes and a greater deficit. Also consider using a quotation about government (e.g., from John F. Kennedy).

Another possibility would be to mention that 'big' government leads to too much power, and "absolute power corrupts absolutely." There are an endless number of possibilities. The key is to choose one line of thinking and present it in a clear manner. {Note how the structure and length of the sentences vary in the example.}

Task 2: Follow a similar approach for tasks two and three. Write down any points you may want to include in your essay which contradict the statement even if you completely agree with it. You should be able to see the other side. If you cannot think of something to challenge the statement, try to think what someone who actively disagrees with the statement would say.

Ex.: i> *Rights of one person begins where another person's rights end: government ensures that happens.*
ii> *National crisis*
iii> *War/draft*

Choose one specific example and elaborate. Take (iii) as a case in point. The writer may use World War II as a specific example. The fact that the government increased its powers by legislating that certain members of the population must go to war (= draft) could be explored. The war prevented the Nazi government from becoming an even greater destructive force and its reign of terror ended. Thus the government expanded its powers for the greater good.

Task 3: For the third task, look back at the ideas you wrote down to address the first two tasks. You should then be able to reconcile the two opposing views. Write down what you think is the key component of your answer to the third task. Remember that you are not expected to solve all the problems in the world. Simply try to find the best way you know to solve the dilemma outlined by the first two tasks. There are no right or wrong answers for this assignment. What is being graded is your reasoning and your ability to express your thoughts.

Ex.: i> *When the survival of the community is endangered*
ii> *Government should govern for the benefit of its citizens*

Prewriting the tasks is not like writing a formal outline. It is simply a way to structure your ideas in order to enable you to write a well-organised essay in 30 minutes. While prewriting might seem like a waste of time, it is the key to helping you complete all three tasks in the time allowed.

Step 3: Organise your notes

Once you have completed the three tasks, you will want to organise and clarify your ideas. This will allow you to examine your ideas before you write and to see how they fit together. You may want to remove some ideas and reformulate others. At this stage, you will decide in which order you will address the three tasks (normally, however, you will keep the order as Tasks 1, 2, 3, respectively). Once you have done this, you will be ready to write the essay. At this point, you will have spent five or six minutes prewriting the tasks. In doing so, you will have created a structure for your essay which will make writing it much easier.

Step 4: Write

When you write, pace yourself. This will be much easier as your notes will provide a framework to work with in writing. You will want to ensure you have a few (about five) minutes to review your masterpiece! Make sure that your essay flows. Use transition words and phrases between your paragraphs. Pay attention to your spelling, punctuation and grammar. Be sure to vary the structure and length of the sentences in your text.

Do not assume that the reader can read your mind! Be explicit in your presentation. Providing a specific, well-illustrated example can impress the marker. And finally, be sure to not digress from the theme of your essay.

Step 5: Proofread

Reread your text. You want to spend your last five minutes proofreading your essay. Look for and correct mistakes and ensure you followed the plan you established as you prewrote the tasks. At this point you want to simply polish your essay.

4.3 Building Your Vocabulary

Clarity of expression makes a GAMSAT Written Communication essay an easy read. On the other hand, it also helps to make an impression on the marker by interweaving words that will add a "wow" factor to your writing. Of course, you don't use "big words" just for the sake of it. You have to make sure that they make sense within the sentence's context. Simply using one or two of these words in your essay will elevate it above many others. Consider making flashcards or audio files on your smartphone with the words you like most to help with repetition.

One way to improve or strengthen your vocabulary skills is to keep a "beautiful-words" notebook. You can build your list by writing down a new word in this notebook every time you find a term that you feel would make your sentences sound more elegant in an essay. The following list is meant to help get you started.

Accoutrement - *(noun)* additional clothing or equipment; accessories

*The Freedom of Information Act is the perfect **accoutrement** to the Bill of Rights.*

Affectation - *(noun)* a display of behaviour or attitude that is artificial or pretentious but meant to impress others. This is different from affection which is a feeling of liking or caring for another person

*The daughter-in-law held her mother-in-law's hand and touched it to her cheek: clearly an **affectation** intending to convey fondness for the old lady who held the family's purse.*

Allegory - *(noun)* the representation of abstract ideas or principles by characters, figures, or events in narrative, dramatic, or pictorial form

*The book, Animal Farm, is an **allegory** of communism and the pitfalls of having a common identity.*

Altruism - *(noun)* a selfless commitment to the service of others

***Altruism** is a rare gift, exemplified by the likes of Mother Teresa and Princess Diana.*

Aphorism - *(noun)* a brief statement containing a general truth or opinion; an adage

*He is the master of Shakespearean **aphorisms**.*

Apocryphal - *(adjective)* of doubtful authority or authenticity but widely made out to be the truth

*Historians are always faced with the challenge of distinguishing authentic happenings from **apocryphal** stories.*

Arcane - *(adjective)* understood by a select few who have the knowledge or interest; mysterious; concealed

*Only real poets can speak the **arcane** language of poetry.*

Bellwether - *(noun)* someone who leads the flock; a person or entity at the forefront of a trend, profession, industry or any other endeavour; trendsetter

*Our biology professor is a **bellwether** of practical science.*

Bifurcate - *(verb)* to divide into two separate branches; forked

*The end of the road **bifurcates**, leading you into two different directions.*

Caveat - *(noun)* a warning or word of caution; specific limits

As comprehensive and eloquent as this policy is, there is still one ***caveat****: it fails to mention where jurisdiction resides.*

Chicanery - *(noun)* the use of tricks to deceive someone (usually to extract money from them)

Chicanery *made him rich and so will be his downfall.*

Circumlocution - *(noun)* an indirect way of conveying one's thoughts and ideas; excessive use of words to express a simple meaning

Laws have become a series of ***circumlocutions****, disconnecting the people from the government and marginalising the poorest of the poor.*

Circumvent - *(verb)* to evade or avoid using strategic or deceptive means; to bypass or go around; to entrap

Individuals who ***circumvent*** *the law are regarded by society as deviants.*

Conundrum - *(noun)* a serious problem with some degree of difficulty; a puzzle, riddle or question asked for the sake of amusement

Through unity and cooperation, social institutions can combat this ***conundrum****.*

Conviviality - *(noun)* a quality marked by good cheer, liveliness and friendliness

His ***conviviality*** *and trustworthiness brought him to the heights of success.*

Cupidity - *(noun)* overwhelming desire (to the point of greed); the excessive urge to possess or covetousness

Human ***cupidity*** *has been subject to much contention in the field of sociology.*

Cynosure - *(noun)* the centre of attention because of its beauty; a guide

An uncompromising policy against corruption is the ***cynosure*** *of the new government.*

Demagogue - *(noun)* a leader who tries to stir up people by appealing to their emotions and prejudices for the purpose of gaining power

Adolf Hitler was the greatest ***demagogue*** *of all time as history itself certifies this claim.*

Discombobulate - (verb) to upset, disconcert; to provoke feelings of confusion or frustration

If you try to ***discombobulate*** *me, I will stop talking to you for months.*

Ebullient - (adjective) energetic, enthusiastic or in high spirits; in a boiling state

*His **ebullient** personality made a lot of people weary except me.*

Eclectic - (adjective) adopting, made up of or combining elements from varying sources; acceptance of or adherence to more than one system of thought, belief, culture or practice

*My friend embraces an **eclectic** way of life, being a Buddhist, a Christian and a Muslim all at the same time.*

Egalitarian - *(adjective)* an assertion and manifestation of or belief in the equality of all people especially in political and socio-economic matters; favouring equality in all aspects

*The French Revolution was a prime example of an uprising fueled by **egalitarian** sentiments.*

Egregious - (adjective) outstandingly bad; notorious

*Such an **egregious** mistake should never be committed again.*

Enfranchise - *(verb)* grant freedom to, as from slavery or servitude; to afford rights or privileges that were previously withheld

*This new system could **enfranchise** and empower women in the labour sector, who feel underrepresented and voiceless.*

Ephemeral - *(adjective)* a temporary condition, situation or state of being; short-lived

*The passing of Princess Diana shows us that no matter how brightly she shined, her glow was still **ephemeral**.*

Epistemology - *(noun)* a system, method or manner of learning; a theory on human knowledge and the process of learning

*From this **epistemology**, he arrived at the conclusion that knowledge and consciousness are distinct entities.*

Equanimity - *(noun)* exuding grace under pressure; composure even in the face of tension

*For the quick delivery of relief services, both public servants and victims must practice **equanimity**.*

Erudite - *(adjective)* characterised by extensive reading or knowledge; well instructed; highly educated or learned

*An **erudite** person like you should go to medical school.*

Excogitate - *(verb)* to devise a plan or think something through; to understand something by carefully studying it

During the meeting, we ***excogitated*** *the best solution to the problem at hand.*

Existential - *(adjective)* relating to or affirming existence; grounded on existence or the experiences of existence; empirical (can be apprehended by the five senses of man, thus, capable of being measured)

Bruno Bettelheim believed that fairy tales that have been passed generation to generation are society's way of helping children deal with ***existential*** *anxieties.*

Expurgate - *(verb)* to omit or modify parts considered indelicate or inappropriate

Economic policies are thoroughly ***expurgated*** *prior to publication.*

Facetious - *(adjective)* characterised by wit and pleasantry; no serious or literal meaning

His ***facetious*** *remarks entertained the crowd.*

Fait accompli - *(noun)* an accomplished and presumably irreversible deed or fact; a done deal

For this bill to be made into law is ***fait accompli****.*

Fatuous - *(adjective)* devoid of intelligence; mindless or foolish

Use your head if you don't want to be a ***fatuous*** *victim of love.*

Gasconade - *(noun)* excessive boasting; a boastful manner of talking

You can actually tell the difference between a sincere memoir and one that's full of ***gasconade****.*

Gerrymander - *(verb)* to divide unfairly and to one's advantage; to manipulate boundaries, as in voting districts, for self-serving reasons

Politicians found guilty of ***gerrymandering*** *will face legal charges and be made to answer to the court of law.*

Halcyon - *(adjective)* pertaining to peaceful, tranquil, undisturbed and happy

The ***halcyon*** *days are gone, replaced by war and strife.*

Hegemony - *(noun)* the dominance or leadership of one social group or nation over others; the pursuit of world domination through aggressive or expansionist acts

Imposing one's political beliefs on other people is a manifestation of ***hegemony****.*

Hubris - *(noun)* an excess of pride or self-confidence

He who falls prey to ***hubris*** *shall fail to see the real meaning of life.*

Hyperbole - *(noun)* a deliberate exaggeration; a figure of speech characterised by extravagant expressions

To say that Helen of Troy's beauty can launch a thousand ships is nothing more than a ***hyperbole****.*

Iconoclast - *(noun)* one who attacks and seeks to overthrow traditional or popular beliefs and ideas of institutions under the assumption of error or irrationality

During the Byzantine era, ***iconoclasts*** *from the Eastern Orthodox faith destroyed religious statues and images that belonged to the Roman Catholic Church.*

Idiosyncratic - *(adjective)* an unusual way in which a particular person behaves or thinks; may also refer to an eccentric feature of something

Dishevelled and unruly hair is ***idiosyncratic*** *of Albert Einstein as purple socks are idiosyncratic to my grandmother.*

Inchoate - *(adjective)* partially but not fully in existence or operation; underdeveloped or incomplete; still at the initial stages

According to the principles of International Law, unless you fully occupy a piece of land, merely discovering it will only give you an ***inchoate*** *title.*

Incognito - *(can be used as a noun, an adjective or an adverb)* without revealing or concealing one's identity in order to avoid notice

The monarch of a 19th century superpower country traveled ***incognito*** *to Australia.*

Irony - *(noun)* an amusing or comical situation that arises from the contradiction of things, especially when expectations are at odds with the resulting reality

*Note: **Irony** is also used in debate and in cross-examination (Socratic irony: where a person who seems to be ignorant, asks questions of someone who appears to be smart only* to *expose that the "smart' person is anything but smart). It is also used in drama (When the sequence of events leads the audience to expect a particular ending but the ending does not conform to expectations, the ending is said to be one of dramatic irony).*

*It is **ironic** that the prankster slipped and fell as he was setting up a prank on someone else.*

Jejune - *(adjective)* not of interest; not distinctive or remarkable in any way; insipid

*The **jejune** lecture caused me to doze off.*

Ken - *(noun)* understanding, perception or knowledge (of an idea or circumstance); to comprehend, recognise or discern

*Maths is a subject that has always been beyond my **ken**.*

Lexicon - *(noun)* a stock of terms used in a particular profession, subject or style; a vocabulary list or a record, collection or inventory of words and terms

*Adorbs and clickbait are now part of the global **lexicon**.*

Magnanimous - *(adjective)* refers to a person's generous and kind nature; may also refer to a lofty and courageous spirit; suggests nobility of feeling and generosity of mind

*Bill Gates was **magnanimous** in his contributions to charity.*

Milieu - *(noun)* social or cultural environment; backdrop or setting

*Our definition of marital union is often dictated by the standards of a particular **milieu**.*

Moiety - *(noun)* one of two (approximately) equal parts; a part of something

*Ethnic tribes comprise one **moiety** of the whole nation.*

Myopic - *(adjective)* lack of discernment or long-range perspective in thinking or planning; inability to act with prudence or foresight; narrow-minded

*Racists and chauvinists have a **myopic** mindset, which can be corrected through immersion in and constant exposure to a pluralist community.*

Nefarious - *(adjective)* wicked in the extreme; promulgates injustice

*I knew he was plotting something **nefarious** when I saw him enter the warehouse.*

Nihilism - *(noun)* complete denial or outright rejection of all established authority, systems and institutions, be it political, economic or social; a preference for anarchy, revolution or absolute destruction

*The Holocaust was a clear manifestation of **nihilism**.*

Obviate - *(verb)* to prevent or eliminate by interception; to render unnecessary

*Studying will **obviate** the risk of getting a low score.*

Oligarchy - *(noun)* a political system governed by a few people, usually of significant wealth and influence; pertains to any other system (economic or social) or institution whereby power is concentrated in the hands of a select group of people

***Oligarchy** is the reason why 75% of our country's population continues to live below the poverty line.*

Ostentatious - *(adjective)* a display of wealth or knowledge that is meant to attract attention admiration or envy; also refers to a fondness for conspicuous and vainglorious and pretentious display

*A peacock, displaying his multicoloured tail feathers to attract a peahen, is not really being **ostentatious**; it assures the peahen that their offspring will be likely as strong and attractive as the peacock, thus ensuring the propagation of their species.*

Paragon - *(noun)* a perfect example of; a model of excellence

*This government is no longer a **paragon** of transparency and accountability.*

Parsimonious - *(adjective)* of or having a thrifty, frugal or stingy disposition

*Experiencing financial failure taught our family to be more **parsimonious**.*

Patrician - *(noun)* a highly educated person of refined upbringing, manners and taste; an aristocrat or someone from a noble or privileged lineage

*The upper echelons of society house individuals with a **patrician** background.*

Pecuniary - *(adjective)* relating to money or monetary transactions

*All **pecuniary** concerns must be directed to the finance officer.*

Pedantic - *(adjective)* learning in an attempt to impress others; bookish or excessively concerned with tiny details

*There's nothing **pedantic** about me joining the Ivy League Debaters Club.*

Pejorative - *(adjective)* has a disparaging, belittling or derogatory impact

*Not to be **pejorative** about it, but the lesson was simply uninteresting.*

Perfidy - *(noun)* intentional treachery or breaking off of trust; any treacherous or dishonest act

Officials found guilty of **perfidy** *should answer for their crimes.*

Pernicious - *(adjective)* results to harm or injury; deadly

*This **pernicious** beast must be tamed before he swallows us all.*

Perspicacious - *(adjective)* having a sharp mental perception; discerning

*Choosing the right candidate requires **perspicacious** judgement.*

Plenary - *(can be used as an adjective or a noun)* fully constituted or complete; a gathering characterised by the presence of all qualified members

*The **plenary** session of the Senate will not start until a quorum is formed.*

Pragmatism - *(noun)* a reasonable and logical way of doing things or thinking about problems that is based on dealing with specific situations instead of on ideals and theories

*Choosing to work from home as a blogger shows the **pragmatism** of a stay-at-home mom of three toddlers: she can earn money while keeping an eye on her children.*

Prevaricate - *(verb)* to create false truths or impressions with the intention to mislead or deceive; to deviate from the truth

*The proletariats believe that the bourgeoisie **prevaricate** their way to the top.*

Probity - *(noun)* honesty, uprightness; with integrity

Citizens are encouraged to vote for political candidates with a proven reputation for ***probity*** *and fairness.*

Proclivity - *(noun)* a natural inclination

The dentist's receptionist has a ***proclivity*** *for discussing trivial details.*

Proficuous - *(adjective)* useful, profitable, advantageous

A ***proficuous*** *turn of events propelled the economy to full recovery.*

Puerile - *(adjective)* displaying a lack of maturity or child-like characteristics; relating to children or youthfulness

What a ***puerile*** *way of looking at things.*

Pusillanimous - *(adjective)* lacking in courage; faint-hearted or cowardly

A person with a ***pusillanimous*** *nature will have a hard time in the military.*

Quotidian - *(adjective)* daily; ordinary; the usual; a common or mundane occurrence

I don't understand why you're so excited when it's just a ***quotidian*** *event.*

Rancor - *(noun)* consumed by bitterness or resentment for a long time

The moment her sister asked for forgiveness, the ***rancor*** *she felt all those years began to melt.*

Renege - *(verb)* to revoke a given promise or commitment

Find another supplier if this one tries to ***renege*** *or demand an unreasonable sum.*

Res Ipsa Loquitur - *(noun)* a legal doctrine referring to situations where an injury was obviously caused by negligence; a legal jargon for "what you see is what you get"

This accident is a case of ***res ipsa loquitor****, seeing that there is not one warning device found anywhere in the vicinity.*

Sangfroid - *(noun)* composure or coolness of mind, sometimes excessive, as shown in dangerous situations or under trying circumstances

*To commit a crime with **sangfroid** is far from normal.*

Sanguine - *(adjective)* confidently optimistic or cheerful; relating to blood or the colour red

*What a **sanguine** face this baby has.*

Sardonic - *(adjective)* bitterly sarcastic; mocking or sneering

*I want to wipe that **sardonic** grin off his face.*

Satire - *(noun)* humour derived from poking fun at social issues and human follies in general

*George Orwell's novel, Animal Farm, is a good example of a political **satire** as it exposes the folly of our notions of equality and sums it up in one phrase: "Everyone is created equal, but some are more equal than others."*

Scintilla - *(noun)* a minute amount; an iota or trace

*Not even a **scintilla** of my fortune will go to that scheming relative.*

Soliloquy - *(noun)* a speech you make or a long diatribe to yourself; a monologue

*She delivered a **soliloquy** in an empty auditorium just to make herself feel better.*

Suffragist - *(noun)* an advocate of the extension of voting rights (especially to women); one who promotes or supports the idea that everyone has the right to vote

*Louisa May Alcott, the author of Little Women, was a famed **suffragist**.*

Susurrus - *(noun)* whispering, humming or rustling sounds; soft murmurs or mutters

*The **susurrus** of leaves was like a lullaby that brought my baby to sleep.*

Tautological - *(adjective)* unnecessary repetition of the same sense in different words; redundant use of words, statements or ideas to the point of vagueness

*This book often makes **tautological** conclusions.*

Temperament - *(noun)* typical behaviour, condition or disposition

*Though he does not have a pleasant **temperament**, he still wins friends wherever he goes.*

Touche - *(interjection)* an expression used to acknowledge a striking point or a clever remark made by another person in a discussion

***Touche**! Your suggestion hit the nail on the head.*

Ubiquitous - *(adjective)* universal, omnipresent or being everywhere; accepted by all

*His name became **ubiquitous** in the current news because of the atrocities exposed during his leadership.*

Unctuous - *(adjective)* unpleasantly and excessively suave; insincere

*Even her charitable works were perceived to be **unctuous** by her disgruntled constituents.*

Usufruct - *(noun)* the right or privilege to enjoy the use and advantages of a property owned by another, not including the destruction or misuse of its substance

*They may not have ownership rights but tenants have **usufruct** rights over their landlord's territory.*

- **Helpful Latin Expressions**

The Western world owes much to the classical language of Latin. Some expressions we use today are borrowed from Latin. Even the terms and concepts that serve as basis for our current systems of government, education, science and philosophy are derived from Latin. For this reason, although no one speaks this language nowadays, Latin lives on as part of English expressions. Here are some of them that might come handy when you write your Written Communication essays. You can choose to use one up to a maximum of two of these phrases in your essay:

A priori - *(adjective)* means something assumed or known even without experience; self-evident

The analysis provided by the speaker mostly stems from ***a priori*** *discernment of one's moral values.*

Ad hoc - *(adjective)* means something that is set up only for this one instance, to address a singular and particular set of circumstances, problem or situation and not as something permanent

The President formed an ***ad hoc*** *committee to assess the rehabilitation needs of places affected by the supertyphoon Haiyan.*

Ad infinitum - *(adverb)* means "endless"; to remember the meaning of this phrase, you only have to remember Buzz Lightyear as this is his catchphrase: "To infinity and beyond."

The nagging wife made it a point to rehearse her husband's faults to his face ***ad infinitum.***

Ad nauseum - *(expression)* signifies a boring and tedious repetition

The doting mother extolled, ***ad nauseam****, the virtues of her beloved son, to anyone who cared to listen.*

Barba tenus sapientes - *(expression)* A man described as barba tenus sapientes is literally said to be "wise as far as his beard". In other words, he might look intelligent but he's actually far from it. This is just one of a number of phrases that show how the Romans associated beards with intelligence, alongside barba non facit philosophum, "a beard does not make a philosopher," and barba crescit caput nescit, meaning "the beard grows, but the head doesn't grow wiser."

Robert doesn't shave off his beard; he thinks it makes him look ***barba tenus sapientes****.*

Bona fide - *(adjective)* means something genuine, honest, authentic and sincere; especially without any intention to deceive or beguile

As per his client's wishes, and against the better judgment of the stockbroker, he made a ***bona fide*** *offer to buy the shares of stock of Enron.*

Brutum fulmen - *(noun)* a harmless or empty threat; literally means "senseless thunderbolt"

When a man who is swaying on his feet from drunkenness tells you he is going to beat you up, you can be sure it's just ***brutus fulmen****.*

Medium-level Importance

Carpe diem - *(expression)* literally means "to seize the day"; conveys the same meaning as "make hay while the sun shines" meaning, seize the opportunities that present themselves. In the movie Dead Poets' Society, the actor Robin Williams played the role of a professor in a prep school who urged his students to "carpe diem" - seize the day.

> *My 70 year-old grandmother, wishing to tick-off items on her bucket list, went bungee jumping – the last thing she said before jumping off was **"Carpe diem!"***

Caveat emptor - *(noun)* a doctrine in both law and business that someone who wishes to buy anything must be aware of the conditions, circumstances and consequences of the purchase as the seller cannot be held responsible unless expressed in a warranty

> *When buying a second-hand car, always look for the car's registration papers and insurance; check that the chassis and engine numbers which appear on the car match the numbers on the registration. After all, this is due diligence because of **caveat emptor**.*

Cogito ergo sum - *(expression or idea)* literally means **"I think, therefore, I am."**; the conclusion reached by the person who wonders whether he exists. In the work by Rene Descartes, the phrase was in French ("Je pense donc je suis."). This phrase became the basis for Western philosophy. For Rene Descartes, existence is self-awareness and self-awareness presumes existence.

Compos mentis - *(adjective)* literally means "of sound mind" ; this phrase usually appears in the negative "non compos mentis" which means "not of a sound mind"; this phrase is often used to describe people who are incompetent to stand trial, to act with legal effect in entering binding contracts

> *The heirs of the 90-year old billionaire went to court asking that he be declared "**non compos mentis**" and therefore, put into their guardianship.*

Coup de grace - *(French expression)* means the final touch or decisive stroke; In art, it is the last brushstroke to a masterpiece. In murder novels, it is the "last strike or the last stroke" meaning, the death blow.

> *The fencer lunges with a **coup de grace** - his foil hits the mark near the heart of his opponent. It was his winning move.*

Medium-level Importance

Cui bono - *(expression)* literally means "Who benefits?"; a rhetorical Latin legal phrase used to imply that whoever appears to have the most to gain from a crime is probably the culprit. More generally, it is used in English to question the meaningfulness or advantages of carrying something out.

*The police detective, all dressed up in the fashion of Sherlock Holmes, turned around most theatrically and said to the relatives of the victim: "**Cui bono**? He who has the most to gain from the crime probably had the strongest motive to commit it."*

De facto - *(noun)* In law and business, it means to exist as a fact even without legal sanction or legal right.

*In Australia, when a man and a woman live together sharing domestic life, they are considered a **de facto** couple and are entitled to the same rights given to married couples.*

De jure - *(noun)* according to law; by legal right

*Adultery is illegal, **de jure**, in many states, but the laws are never enforced.*

De novo - *(adverb)* used in English to mean "anew" or "afresh"

*When one appeals a lower court decision, the appellate court usually reviews the evidence **de novo**.*

Dum spiro spero - *(expression or motto)* literally means, "While I breathe, I hope."; the English equivalent is "Hope springs eternal."

*My grandmother, on a hospital bed after suffering a stroke, said to the doctor who told her that she might not be able to drive a car anymore: **"Dum spiro spero."***

E pluribus unum - *(expression or motto)* literally means "out of many, one"

*The Latin phrase "**E pluribus unum**" appears on the seal of the United States as it is the official motto of the United States of America, signifying the federal system of government.*

Errare humanum est - *(expression)* literally means "to err is human"; It means that it is expected for mortal men to make mistakes. This harks back to the Biblical story of the first man, Adam, and how he and his wife, Eve, fell into sin. The rest of humanity which was begotten of them, therefore inherited the tendency to err, to make mistakes and to sin. The entire phrase is: "Errare humanum est, et ignoscere divinum." (Translated: To err is human, and to forgive, divine.")

Félix cupla - *(noun)* literally a "happy fault"; an apparent mistake or disaster that actually ends up having surprisingly beneficial consequences

> *Losing my job when I was laid off, although quite a stressful experience, turned out to be a **félix culpa** since I started a business, which is now quite profitable.*

Imperium in emperio - *(noun)* meaning "an empire within an empire"; can be used literally to refer to a self-governing state confined within a larger one; or to a rebellious state fighting for independence from another; or, more figuratively, to a department or a group of workers in an organisation who, despite appearing to work for themselves, are still answerable to an even larger corporation.

> *The IT Department at our office is an **imperium in imperio**: it is made up of techie geeks who work independently, often ignoring the office dress code and the designated office hours.*

Je ne sais quoi - *(noun)* This is actually French phrase which literally means "I don't know what"; its English equivalent is 'a certain something'; refers to an innate quality of a person or thing that makes them attractive but which cannot be quantified, articulated, or put into words

> *To be a supermodel, it is not enough to be merely tall or beautifully proportioned; one also needs to have a presence, a certain **je ne sais quoi**.*

Mea culpa - *(expression)* literally means "the fault is mine"; it is the Latin equivalent of a plea of guilty in court; also a form of apology

> *The witness exclaimed, "**Mea culpa!**" when the opposing lawyer showed her a discrepancy in her recollection of events.*

Modus operandi - *(noun)* often used to describe a signature move or signature moves of criminals

> *Most internet scammers have the same* ***modus operandi****: they send you an email informing you that you have won several thousand dollars but in order to receive the entire amount, you are to deposit a certain smaller amount to "verify" your account and whereabouts.*

Non sequitur - *(noun)* an illogical conclusion; the opposite of "et sequitur" which means "and so on and so forth"; usually indicates that there is a logical gap between two propositions

> *Just because I agreed to go out on one date with you, it doesn't mean I love you or I want to marry you – that is* ***non sequitur****.*

Panem et circensēs - *(noun)* means "bread and circuses"; refers to the basic needs and desires - i.e., food and entertainment - to keep a person happy

> *In order to keep the Roman citizens from becoming an unruly mob, the emperors took it as their political duty to provide them with* ***panem et circensēs*** *to keep them quiet and compliant.*

Persona non grata - *(noun)* literally means "an unwelcome person"; the term is primarily used of diplomatic officials from other countries when they have committed crimes in a host country and are expelled from that host country

> *Even when he was accused of sexually harassing his personal assistant, the attaché could not be criminally charged but he was declared "****persona non grata****" and he left for his home country.*

Quid pro quo - *(noun)* literally means "this for that"; the original phrase signifies an exchange of things with equivalent value; the English equivalent is "tit for tat" signifying an equivalent retaliation;

> *The serial killer Hannibal Lester refused to answer the FBI agent's questions unless the FBI agent herself answers his questions regarding her personal life; he told her "****Quid pro quo****, Clarisse."*

Semper Fi - *(noun)* This is the motto of the US Marines which means "Always faithful" or "Always keep the faith". This motto comes with a twin "Marines leave no man behind." This signifies the camaraderie in arms of the Marines that in battle, at great risk to themselves, they will bring home the men with whom they fought side by side, be they dead or alive. It also signifies that Marines will always be faithful to their oath to uphold their nation's defense.

Sine qua non - *(noun)* something you cannot do without; in law, it is an absolute condition, that is, it is a condition that must be met before entering into a privilege or a right

*When Sara's grandmother bequeathed to her one million dollars in her will, she made Sara's marriage a **sine qua non** to the inheritance.*

Status quo - *(noun)* In law, this phrase is used as "status quo ante" which means, the status or state of affairs prior to the present controversy; in everyday language, the term "status quo" means the actual state of affairs in the present. The best way to remember this phrase is by calling to mind the Disney movie High School Musical:

*The popular girl, Sharpe Adams, was opposed to the basketball athletes and Maths wizards joining the drama club and the musical so she sang, "stick to the **status quo**."*

Tempus fugit - *(expression)* literally means "time flies"; in English, the phrase "time flies when you're having fun" comes from the Latin phrase 'tempus fugit'.

Veni, vidi, vici - *(expression or motto)* This is what Julius Ceasar said when he reported to the Roman Senate after he conquered the Gauls (of France) "I came, I saw, I conquered."

Verbatim - *(can be used as adverb or adjective)* means "word for word"; a precise and exact quote of what someone said

*The senator said to the reporter who was interviewing him: "You can quote me on that, in fact, quote me **verbatim**, why don't you?"*

Veto - *(can be used as noun or verb)* the political power to single-handedly stop or make void a law

*The new immigration bill passed by a slim margin in Congress, but the President is likely to **veto** it.*

Vox populi - *(noun)* literally means "the voice of the people"; refers to public opinion

*When elected viva voce by the Roman mob, this is what the elected official says when he accepts the elected position "**vox populi**, vox dei" which means, God has spoken through the people.*

4.4 Practice Materials

It is great to know the structure, as previously described, for Task A and Task B. However, you must practice generating ideas and expressing yourself.

Practice Problems
• Brainstorm using famous quotes (WC 4.5)
• Generate thesis statements using sets of quotes (WC 4.6)
• ACER's Automatic Scoring for Written Communication
• Gold Standard (GS) Essay-correction Service
Full-length Practice Tests
• 5 GS Online GAMSAT Practice Tests
• GAMSAT Heaps: 15 Full-length Practice Tests for the GAMSAT (this includes the 5 GS tests)
• ACER Materials

Currently, your real GAMSAT Written Communication essays are scored by 3 human beings and, if necessary, a fourth as an arbiter. ACER offers a paid, automated, essay-scoring service. At the time of printing, the system can correct 16 essays (8 prompts for Task A and 8 for Task B) for less than the price of a single ACER practice test (AUD $20; £11; €13). Incredibly, most students (*of course, not all students*) have found that ACER's service accurately predicted their real exam score in Written Communication, within a small margin of error. Automation scores again!

Gold Standard's Essay-correction Service does not have access to the extensive data that ACER has to be able to standardise GAMSAT scores from 3-4 markers. You cannot count on accurate predictions but you can count on personalised, helpful comments from an expert.

You can submit 2 typed essays at any time of the year except within 7 days of any GAMSAT sitting, not beyond 2 years of purchase, for the original owner only, consistent with our Terms of Use. This bonus offer is not transferable. On average, students receive their scored essays - including critiques - within one week.

Also note: You can submit essays in response to any prompts. You can use prompts in this book, or prompts in your account at gamsat-prep.com, or prompts from ACER's materials or yet another source. You must submit your typed essays in your account after registration here:

www.gamsat-prep.com/gamsat-essays-written-communication/

Note: If you purchased this textbook or the eBook directly from www.gamsat-prep.com, then your online access is automated.

Good luck!

High-level Importance

4.5 Advice on How to Generate Ideas

Many candidates struggle in generating their initial ideas for an essay. One possible root cause may be a difficulty in comprehending the idea expressed in a quotation. In most cases, you will simply not know enough about the topic. By writing a timed essay, and then revising it by doing research outside of exam conditions, you will grow your body of knowledge. This body of knowledge is what separates the very high achievers from the median in Written Communication.

As your knowledge builds, you may still experience issues attempting to piece together your arguments and evidence. One way to address this problem is by having a ready set of guide questions that you can actively ask yourself while you consider a given quotation. The following are some of these possible questions:

Main idea/Introduction:

1. What is the quotation talking about?
2. What is its main point?

Thesis/Body:

1. What is my immediate thought or reaction to the quotation?
2. What is the significant issue / first-hand experience that I can relate to my thesis?
3. Check for focus and relevance: How does it connect to the view reflected by the quotation?

Antithesis/Body:

1. What opinion or situation can I recall, based on knowledge or experience, that will counter my initial view in the thesis?
2. Check again for focus and relevance: How does it connect to the central idea presented in the quotation?

Synthesis/Conclusion:

1. How do I reconcile the two opposing views with my thesis?
2. How do I connect these views in my present socio-cultural or interpersonal context?

We have placed 50 quotations for you to work through. Half for Writing Task A and the other half for Writing Task B. Please consider re-reading WC 4.2.5 and WC 4.2.6. Your aim is to quickly key in on the idea being presented and generate ideas in point form in less than 5 minutes. Frankly, your efficiency should increase in the last 10 essays in each section. Do not try to complete all the exercises in one sitting.

You can discuss the way you structured your essay with other students in our Forum.

4.5.1 Writing Task A Quotations

1. Let us never negotiate out of fear. But let us never fear to negotiate.

   John F. Kennedy

   Thesis ____________________
   Antithesis ____________________
   Synthesis ____________________

2. We live in a moment in history where change is so speeded up that we begin to see the present only when it is already disappearing.

   R.D. Laing

   Thesis ____________________
   Antithesis ____________________
   Synthesis ____________________

3. All diplomacy is a continuation of war by other means.

   Chou En-Lai

   Thesis ____________________
   Antithesis ____________________
   Synthesis ____________________

4. It is better that ten guilty persons escape than one innocent suffer.

   William Blackstone

   Thesis ____________________
   Antithesis ____________________
   Synthesis ____________________

5. Money is like the sixth sense without which you cannot make a complete use of the other five.

   W. Somerset Maugham

   Thesis ____________________
   Antithesis ____________________
   Synthesis ____________________

6. That man is richest whose pleasures are the cheapest.

   Henry David Thoreau

   Thesis ____________________
   Antithesis ____________________
   Synthesis ____________________

7. The technologies which have had the most profound effects on human life are usually simple.

Freeman Dyson

Thesis ______________________________
Antithesis ______________________________
Synthesis ______________________________

8. The great growling engine of change - technology.

Alvin Toffler

Thesis ______________________________
Antithesis ______________________________
Synthesis ______________________________

9. Ability is a poor man's wealth.

John Wooden

Thesis ______________________________
Antithesis ______________________________
Synthesis ______________________________

10. The mother of revolution and crime is poverty.

Aristotle quotes

Thesis ______________________________
Antithesis ______________________________
Synthesis ______________________________

11. It is better to be defeated on principle than to win on lies.

Arthur Calwell

Thesis ______________________________
Antithesis ______________________________
Synthesis ______________________________

12. Those who make peaceful revolution impossible will make violent revolution inevitable.

John F. Kennedy

Thesis ______________________________
Antithesis ______________________________
Synthesis ______________________________

13. Injustice anywhere is a threat to justice everywhere.

Martin Luther King, Jr.

Thesis ______________________________
Antithesis ______________________________
Synthesis ______________________________

14. ...government of the people, by the people, for the people, shall not perish from the earth.

Abraham Lincoln

Thesis ______________________________
Antithesis ______________________________
Synthesis ______________________________

15. In the long-run every Government is the exact symbol of its People, with their wisdom and unwisdom.

Thomas Carlyle

Thesis ____________________

Antithesis ____________________

Synthesis ____________________

16. The cost of liberty is less than the price of repression.

W. E. B. Du Bois

Thesis ____________________

Antithesis ____________________

Synthesis ____________________

17. I have to follow them, I am their leader.

Alexandre-Auguste Ledru-Rollin

Thesis ____________________

Antithesis ____________________

Synthesis ____________________

18. I would rather be exposed to the inconveniences attending too much liberty than those attending too small a degree of it.

Thomas Jefferson

Thesis ____________________

Antithesis ____________________

Synthesis ____________________

19. Those who expect to reap the blessings of freedom, must, like men, undergo the fatigues of supporting it.

Thomas Jefferson

Thesis ____________________

Antithesis ____________________

Synthesis ____________________

20. The only way to make sure people you agree with can speak is to support the rights of people you don't agree with.

Eleanor Holmes Norton

Thesis ____________________

Antithesis ____________________

Synthesis ____________________

21. I disapprove of what you say, but I will defend to the death your right to say it.

Voltaire

Thesis ____________________

Antithesis ____________________

Synthesis ____________________

22. He that would make his own liberty secure must guard even his enemy from oppression.

Thomas Paine

Thesis ______
Antithesis ______
Synthesis ______

23. War settles nothing.

Dwight D. Eisenhower

Thesis ______
Antithesis ______
Synthesis ______

24. You can't hold a man down without staying down with him.

Booker T. Washington

Thesis ______
Antithesis ______
Synthesis ______

25. Men prize the thing ungained, more than it is.

Shakespeare

Thesis ______
Antithesis ______
Synthesis ______

4.5.2 Writing Task B Quotations

1. It is amazing how complete the delusion that beauty is goodness.

Leo Tolstoy

Introduction ______
Body ______
Conclusion ______

2. Whether you think you can or think you can't - you are right.

Henry Ford

Introduction ______
Body ______
Conclusion ______

3. From the deepest desires often come the deadliest hate.

Socrates

Introduction ______________________________

Body ______________________________

Conclusion ______________________________

4. The error of youth is to believe that intelligence is a substitute for experience, while the error of age is to believe that experience is a substitute for intelligence.

Lyman Bryson

Introduction ______________________________

Body ______________________________

Conclusion ______________________________

5. Conform and be dull.

James Frank Dobie

Introduction ______________________________

Body ______________________________

Conclusion ______________________________

6. You can stay young as long as you can learn, acquire new habits and suffer contradictions.

Marie von Ebner-Eschenbach

Introduction ______________________________

Body ______________________________

Conclusion ______________________________

7. Hatred is the coward's revenge for being intimidated.

George Bernard Shaw

Introduction ______________________________

Body ______________________________

Conclusion ______________________________

8. The young always have the same problem – how to rebel and conform at the same time. They have now solved this by defying their parents and copying one another.

Quentin Crisp

Introduction ______________________________

Body ______________________________

Conclusion ______________________________

9. Youth is the best time to be rich, and the best time to be poor.

Euripides

Introduction ______________________________

Body ______________________________

Conclusion ______________________________

10. Some people say they haven't yet found themselves. But the self is not something one finds; it is something one creates.

Thomas Szasz

Introduction ____________________
Body ____________________
Conclusion ____________________

11. My youth is escaping without giving me anything it owes me.

Ivy Compton-Burnett

Introduction ____________________
Body ____________________
Conclusion ____________________

12. You can't get rid of poverty by giving people money.

P.J. O'Rourke

Introduction ____________________
Body ____________________
Conclusion ____________________

13. Nobody can make you feel inferior without your consent.

Eleanor Roosevelt

Introduction ____________________
Body ____________________
Conclusion ____________________

14. Youth is something very new: twenty years ago no one mentioned it.

Coco Chanel

Introduction ____________________
Body ____________________
Conclusion ____________________

15. There are three things extremely hard: steel, a diamond, and to know one's self.

Benjamin Franklin

Introduction ____________________
Body ____________________
Conclusion ____________________

16. Comedy is the last refuge of the nonconformist mind.

Edward Albee

Introduction ____________________
Body ____________________
Conclusion ____________________

17. When she stopped conforming to the conventional picture of femininity she finally began to enjoy being a woman.

Betty Naomi Friedan

Introduction ______________________________
Body ______________________________
Conclusion ______________________________

18. When you can't remember why you're hurt, that's when you're healed.

Jane Fonda

Introduction ______________________________
Body ______________________________
Conclusion ______________________________

19. Laughter is the shortest distance between two people.

Victor Borge

Introduction ______________________________
Body ______________________________
Conclusion ______________________________

20. In prison, those things withheld from and denied to the prisoner become precisely what he wants most of all.

Eldridge Cleaver

Introduction ______________________________
Body ______________________________
Conclusion ______________________________

21. People travel to wonder at the height of mountains, at the huge waves of the sea, at the long courses of rivers, at the vast compass of the ocean, at the circular motion of the stars, and they pass themselves by without wondering.

St. Augustine

Introduction ______________________________
Body ______________________________
Conclusion ______________________________

22. Ask the young. They know everything.

Joseph Joubert

Introduction ______________________________
Body ______________________________
Conclusion ______________________________

23. A sense of humor is a major defense against minor troubles.

Mignon McLaughlin

Introduction ______________________________
Body ______________________________
Conclusion ______________________________

24. If the misery of the poor be caused not by the laws of nature, but by our institutions, great is our sin.
Charles Darwin

Introduction ______________________________
Body ______________________________
Conclusion ______________________________

25. They can't hurt you unless you let them.
Multiple attributions

Introduction ______________________________
Body ______________________________
Conclusion ______________________________

4.6 Exercises for Developing a Logical Response

Some candidates do not have much of a problem understanding quotations. However, they may find difficulty in identifying the central theme of the different quotations. We have prepared 20 sets of 5 comments each as supplementary exercises - 10 for Writing Task A and the remaining 10 for Writing Task B.

You may want to revise WC 4.2.1 before going through these exercises. You may also use the templates found in WC 4.11 as guides for developing your essays.

Note: These are important mental exercises to further develop your skill to express your ideas clearly. Another bonus to these exercises, is that you are creating notes that you can regularly consult in the weeks before the real exam. During that period, you can keep reliving the process of idea-generation and expression across a multitude of themes which increases your preparedness for the real exam.

4.6.1 Writing Task A Exercises

Exercise 1:

Comment 1

Without censorship, things can get terribly confused in the public mind.

William Westmoreland

* * * * *

Comment 2

I don't believe in censorship, but I do believe that an artist has to take some moral responsibility for what he or she is putting out there.

Tom Petty

* * * * *

Comment 3

If you have to be careful because of oppression and censorship, this pressure produces diamonds.

Tatyana Tolstaya

* * * * *

Comment 4

The most dangerous untruths are truths moderately distorted.

Georg Christoph Lichtenberg

* * * * *

Comment 5

To forbid us anything is to make us have a mind for it.

Michel de Montaigne

Topic:____

Socio-cultural Theme/Issue: ______________________________

Thesis Statement:_____________________________________

Exercise 2:

Comment 1

Only when the last tree has died and the last river been poisoned and the last fish been caught will we realise we cannot eat money.

Indian Cree Proverb

* * * * *

Comment 2

Environmentally friendly cars will soon cease to be an option . . . they will become a necessity.

Fujio Cho

* * * * *

Comment 3

I would feel more optimistic about a bright future for man if he spent less time proving that he can outwit Nature and more time tasting her sweetness and respecting her seniority.

Elwyn Brooks White

Comment 4

Every human has a fundamental right to an environment of quality that permits a life of dignity and well-being.

* * * * *

Comment 5

After one look at this planet any visitor from outer space would say "I want to see the manager".

William S. Burroughs

Topic:____

Socio-cultural Theme/Issue: ______________________________

Thesis Statement:__________________________________

Exercise 3:

Comment 1

My personal opinion (not speaking for IBM) is that DRM [Digital Rights Management] is stupid, because it can never be effective, and it takes away existing rights of the consumer.

David Safford

* * * * *

Comment 2

Digital files cannot be made uncopyable, any more than water can be made not wet.

Bruce Schneier

* * * * *

Comment 3

Trusted systems presume that the consumer is dishonest.

Mark J. Stefik

* * * * *

Comment 4

Hoaxes use weaknesses in human behavior to ensure they are replicated and distributed. In other words, hoaxes prey on the Human Operating System.

Stewart Kirkpatrick

* * * * *

Comment 5

It's baffling to me that the content industries don't look at the experience of the software industry in the 80's, when copy protection on software was widely tried, and just as widely rejected by consumers.

Tim O'Reilly

Topic:____

Socio-cultural Theme/Issue: ______________________________

Thesis Statement:___________________________________

Exercise 4:

Comment 1

If the past cannot teach the present and the father cannot teach the son, then history need not have bothered to go on, and the world has wasted a great deal of time.

Russell Hoban

* * * * *

Comment 2

The best of my education has come from the public library . . . my tuition fee is a bus fare and once in a while, five cents a day for an overdue book. You don't need to know very much to start with, if you know the way to the public library.

Lesley Conger

* * * * *

Comment 3

He who opens a school door, closes a prison.

Victor Hugo

* * * * *

Comment 4

Education is an ornament in prosperity and a refuge in adversity.

Aristotle

* * * * *

Comment 5

Education... has produced a vast population able to read but unable to distinguish what is worth reading.

G. M. Trevelyan

Topic:____

Socio-cultural Theme/Issue: ______________________________

Thesis Statement:__________________________________

Exercise 5:

Comment 1

Technology makes it possible for people to gain control over everything, except over technology.

John Tudor

* * * * *

Comment 2

Humanity is acquiring all the right technology for all the wrong reasons.

R. Buckminster Fuller

* * * * *

Comment 3

If it keeps up, man will atrophy all his limbs but the push-button finger.

Frank Lloyd Wright

* * * * *

Comment 4

The real danger is not that computers will begin to think like men, but that men will begin to think like computers.

Sydney J. Harris

* * * * *

Comment 5

It has become appallingly obvious that our technology has exceeded our humanity.

Albert Einstein

Topic:____

Socio-cultural Theme/Issue: ______________________________

Thesis Statement:____________________________________

Exercise 6:

Comment 1

Government, even in its best state, is but a necessary evil; in its worst state, an intolerable one.

Thomas Paine

* * * * *

Comment 2

The worst thing in this world, next to anarchy, is government.

Henry Ward Beecher

* * * * *

Comment 3

Freedom is when the people can speak, democracy is when the government listens.

Alastair Farrugia

* * * * *

Comment 4

Good government is no substitute for self-government.

Mahatma Gandhi

* * * * *

Comment 5

Every civilised society needs a government that will protect the people's lives and rights to liberty and property.

Topic:______________________________

Socio-cultural Theme/Issue: ________________________

Thesis Statement:____________________________

Exercise 7:

Comment 1

Globalisation has changed us into a company that searches the world, not just to sell or to source, but to find intellectual capital – the world's best talents and greatest ideas.

Jack Welch

* * * * *

Comment 2

It has been said that arguing against globalisation is like arguing against the laws of gravity.

Kofi Annan

* * * * *

Comment 3

Globalisation means we have to re-examine some of our ideas, and look at ideas from other countries, from other cultures, and open ourselves to them.

Herbie Hancock

* * * * *

Comment 4

Globalisation has created this interlocking fragility. At no time in the history of the universe has the cancellation of a Christmas order in New York meant layoffs in China.

Nassim Nicholas Taleb

* * * * *

Comment 5

Globalisation by the way of McDonald's and KFC has captured the hearts, the minds, and from what I can see through the window, the growing bellies of the folks here.

Raquel Cepeda

Topic:____

Socio-cultural Theme/Issue: ________________________________

Thesis Statement:______________________________________

Exercise 8:

Comment 1

Capitalism is an organised system to guarantee that greed becomes the primary force of our economic system and allows the few at the top to get very wealthy and has the rest of us riding around thinking we can be that way, too.

Michael Moore

* * * * *

Comment 2

I am opposing a social order in which it is possible for one man who does absolutely nothing that is useful to amass a fortune of hundreds of millions of dollars, while millions of men and women who work all the days of their lives secure barely enough for a wretched existence.

Eugene V. Debs

* * * * *

Comment 3

Capitalism tries for a delicate balance: It attempts to work things out so that everyone gets just enough stuff to keep them from getting violent and trying to take other people's stuff.

George Carlin

* * * * *

Comment 4

Today's consumers are not opposed to companies making a profit; they want more empathic, enlightened corporations that seek a balance between profit and purpose.

* * * * *

Comment 5

You cannot help the poor by destroying the rich. . . You cannot lift the wage earner by pulling the wage payer down . . . You cannot help people permanently by doing for them, what they could and should do for themselves.

Abraham Lincoln

Topic:____

Socio-cultural Theme/Issue: ______________________________

Thesis Statement:__________________________________

Exercise 9:

Comment 1

People demand freedom of speech as a compensation for the freedom of thought which they seldom use.

Soren Kierkegaard

* * * * *

Comment 2

Freedom of speech means freedom for those who you despise, and freedom to express the most despicable views.

Alan Dershowitz

* * * * *

Comment 3

The Internet's like one big bathroom wall with a lot of people who anonymously can say really mean things.

Zooey Deschanel

* * * * *

Comment 4

If liberty means anything at all, it means the right to tell people what they do not want to hear.

George Orwell

Comment 5

Freedom of speech does not protect you from the consequences of saying stupid shit.

Jim C. Hines

Topic:____

Socio-cultural Theme/Issue: ______________________________

Thesis Statement:___________________________________

Exercise 10:

Comment 1

Helping those who have been struck by unforseeable misfortunes is fundamentally different from making dependency a way of life.

Thomas Sowell

* * * * *

Comment 2

Dependency is death to initiative, to risk-taking and opportunity. It's time to stop the spread of government dependency and fight it like the poison it is.

Mitt Romney

* * * * *

Comment 3

We must promote upward mobility, starting with solutions that speak to our broken education system, broken immigration policy, and broken safety net programs that foster dependency instead of helping people get back on their feet.

Paul Ryan

* * * * *

Comment 4

Once you go on welfare, it changes you. Even if you get off welfare, you never escape the stigma that you were a charity case.

Jeannette Walls

* * * * *

Comment 5

I do not believe that the power and duty of the General Government ought to be extended to the relief of individual suffering which is in no manner properly related to the public service or benefit.

Grover Cleveland

Topic:____

Socio-cultural Theme/Issue: ______________________________

Thesis Statement:__________________________________

4.6.2 Writing Task B Exercises

Exercise 1:

Comment 1

A man's growth is seen in the successive choirs of his friends.

Ralph Waldo Emerson

* * * * *

Comment 2

Friendship is a single soul dwelling in two bodies.

Aristotle

* * * * *

Comment 3

I have friends in overalls whose friendship I would not swap for the favor of the kings of the world.

Thomas Edison

* * * * *

Comment 4

The bird a nest, the spider a web, man friendship.

William Blake

* * * * *

Comment 5

True friends stab you in the front.

Oscar Wilde

Topic:____

Personal/Social Issues: ________________________________

Thesis Statement:___________________________________

Exercise 2:

Comment 1

In every man's heart there is a secret nerve that answers to the vibrations of beauty.

Christopher Morley

* * * * *

Comment 2

I see beauty as the grace point between what hurts and what heals, between the shadow of tragedy and the light of joy. I find beauty in my scars.

* * * * *

Comment 3

What makes the desert beautiful is that somewhere it hides a well..

The Little Prince, Antoine de Saint Exupery

* * * * *

Comment 4

When you have only two pennies left in the world, buy a loaf of bread with one, and a lily with the other.

Chinese Proverb

* * * * *

Comment 5

We ascribe beauty to that which is simple; which has no superfluous parts; which exactly answers its end; which stands related to all things; which is the mean of many extremes.

Ralph Waldo Emerson

Topic:____

Personal/Social Issues: ________________________________

Thesis Statement:__________________________________

Exercise 3:

Comment 1

Where love rules, there is no will to power; and where power predominates, there love is lacking. The one is the shadow of the other.

Carl Jung

* * * * *

Comment 2

Contrary to Pascal's saying, we don't love qualities, we love persons; sometimes by reason of their defects as well as of their qualities.

Jacques Martain

* * * * *

Comment 3

Love is like racing across the frozen tundra on a snowmobile which flips over, trapping you underneath. At night, the ice-weasels come.

Tom Robbins

* * * * *

Comment 4

If somebody says, "I love you", to me, I feel as though I had a pistol pointed at my head. What can anybody reply under such conditions but that which the pistol-holder requires? "I love you, too".

Kurt Vonnegut, Jr.

* * * * *

Comment 5

They do not love that do not show their love. The course of true love never did run smooth. Love is a familiar. Love is a devil. There is no evil angel but Love.

William Shakespeare

Topic:____

Personal/Social Issues: ________________________________

Thesis Statement:___________________________________

Exercise 4:

Comment 1

Experience is not what happens to you. It is what you do with what happens to you.

Aldous Huxley

* * * * *

Comment 2

It is not only for what we do that we are held responsible, but also for what we do not do.

Moliere

* * * * *

Comment 3

Experience is a hard teacher because she gives the test first, the lesson afterward.

Vernon Law

* * * * *

Comment 4

Life teaches none but those who study it.

V. O. Kliuchevsky

* * * * *

Comment 5

Experience is a great advantage. The problem is that when you get the experience, you're too damned old to do anything about it.

Jimmy Connors

Topic:____

Personal/Social Issues: ________________________________

Thesis Statement:___________________________________

Exercise 5:

Comment 1

The road of excess leads to the palace of wisdom.

William Blake

* * * * *

Comment 2

One's first step in wisdom is to question everything - and one's last is to come to terms with everything.

Georg Christoph Lichtenberg

* * * * *

Comment 3

Wisdom begins at the end.

Daniel Webster

* * * * *

Comment 4

The wisest mind has something yet to learn.

George Santayana

* * * * *

Comment 5

He who devotes sixteen hours a day to hard study may become at sixty as wise as he thought himself at twenty.

Mary Wilson Little

Topic:____

Personal/Social Issues: ________________________________

Thesis Statement:__________________________________

Exercise 6:

Comment 1

Heroes are ordinary people who make themselves extraordinary.

Gerard Way

* * * * *

Comment 2

Anyone who does anything to help a child in his life is a hero to me.

Fred Rogers

* * * * *

Comment 3

I would describe a hero as a person who has no fear of life, who can face life squarely.

Alexander Lowen

* * * * *

Comment 4

Those who say that we're in a time when there are no heroes, they just don't know where to look.

Ronald Reagan

* * * * *

Comment 5

The real hero is always a hero by mistake; he dreams of being an honest coward like everybody else.

Umberto Eco

Topic:____

Personal/Social Issues: ________________________________

Thesis Statement:___________________________________

Exercise 7:

Comment 1

Forgiveness is a virtue of the brave.

Indira Gandhi

* * * * *

Comment 2

It is easier to forgive an enemy than to forgive a friend.

William Blake

* * * * *

Comment 3

You can make up a quarrel, but it will always show where it was patched.

Edgar Watson Howe

* * * * *

Comment 4

To err is human; to forgive, divine.

Alexander Pope

* * * * *

Comment 5

There is no revenge so complete as forgiveness.

Josh Billings

Topic:____

Personal/Social Issues: ____

Thesis Statement:____

Exercise 8:

Comment 1

The worst loneliness is not to be comfortable with yourself.

Mark Twain

* * * * *

Comment 2

Solitude is the profoundest fact of the human condition. Man is the only being who knows he is alone.

Octavio Paz

* * * * *

Comment 3

Loneliness is a barrier that prevents one from uniting with the inner self.

Carl Rogers

* * * * *

Comment 4

At the innermost core of all loneliness is a deep and powerful yearning for union with one's lost self.

Brendan Francis

* * * * *

Comment 5

To dare to live alone is the rarest courage; since there are many who had rather meet their bitterest enemy in the field, than their own hearts in their closet.

Charles Caleb Colton

Topic:____

Personal/Social Issues: ____

Thesis Statement:____

Exercise 9:

Comment 1

If you want creative workers, give them enough time to play.

John Cleese

* * * * *

Comment 2

There is a time for work and there is a time for play. Don't ever mix both.

* * * * *

Comment 3

This is the real secret of life - to be completely engaged with what you are doing in the here and now. And instead of calling it work, realise it is play.

Alan Wilson Watts

* * * * *

Comment 4

There is virtue in work and there is virtue in rest. Use both and overlook neither.

Alan Cohen

* * * * *

Comment 5

You can discover more about a person in an hour of play than in a year of conversation.

Plato

Topic:____

Personal/Social Issues: ________________________________

Thesis Statement:___________________________________

Exercise 10:

Comment 1

Attitude is a little thing that makes a big difference.

Winston Churchill

* * * * *

Comment 2

Excellence is not a skill. It is an attitude.

Ralph Marston

* * * * *

Comment 3

Our attitude towards others determines their attitude towards us.

Earl Nightingale

* * * * *

Comment 4

You cannot change what has already happened - but your attitude can.

* * * * *

Comment 5

Weakness of attitude becomes weakness of character.

Albert Einstein

Topic:____

Personal/Social Issues: ______________________________

Thesis Statement:____________________________________

4.7 The Scoring Key

Your score in the Written Communication section will mostly be based on how you present your ideas. Although technical issues - like occasional grammar and spelling errors - essentially influence the quality of your writing, these are only assessed relative to the effectiveness of your general response. Your personal stand and attitude towards the subject matter will not be part of the assessment. The following are two primary criteria on which Written Communication is assessed: thought and content, and organisation and expression.

Thought and content refers to the substance of your ideas in response to a text. The GAMSAT gives emphasis on generative thinking, which is basically about generating values and innovative ideas in your writing within the thirty minutes per essay time limit. The way you effectively carry out your thoughts and feelings as responses to the task give weight to this criterion.

Organisation and expression is how you develop those fresh ideas in a logical and coherent manner. Control of language, i.e., grammar and fluency, is an inherent consideration in the assessment. However, your skills in this area will only be secondary to the overall content of your response.

Most papers are evaluated on common scoring descriptions. It is advisable that you ask someone to correct your essay to get a general idea. Have this person go through the following guide. Please be reminded that this is not endorsed by ACER and should only be considered as a guide to provide you with a general idea of the process.

Typical Essay Grade	Characteristics of a Paper	Estimated Conversion to a GAMSAT Score
6/6	Thought and content shows clear and coherent transitions of ideas. The writer stays focussed on the subject or issue. There is evidence of a logical build-up of arguments (i.e., normally just Task A but possibly Task B) or reflective discussion (i.e., Task B). Command of the language is excellent.	≥ 72
5/6	Writing shows clarity of ideas with a certain extent of complexity. The argument stays focussed on the issue while main ideas are well-developed. Control of the language is strong.	65–71

Typical Essay Grade	Characteristics of a Paper	Estimated Conversion to a GAMSAT Score
4/6	The essay observes clarity of thought and some depth in ideas. There is also a development of major points and some focus. Control of the language is adequate.	58–64
3/6	There is evidence of some problems with integration and transition of ideas. Major ideas need to be organised and discussed clearly. Errors in grammar and mechanics are evident.	51–57
2/6	Thought and content are disorganised and unclear. There is a lack of logical organisation of main ideas. There are numerous errors in grammar, usage and structure.	44–50
1/6	The essay shows a lack of comprehension about the writing task. There is no development and organisation of ideas. Poor handling of the language prevents the reader from following the points of the writer.	≤ 43

In the next section (WC 4.8), you will find a couple of corrected Written Communication essays and later, in WC 4.9, we will present some excellent essays for your perusal. Also, we have placed dozens of Written Communication essays online that were corrected using the Gold Standard (GS) Essay-correction Service. Of course, you can also leave comments at GAMSAT-prep.com/forum.

4.8 Sample Corrected Essays

In this section, you will find two response essays with corresponding comments. If you wish, use this as yet another exercise. Time yourself (30 minutes) and create an essay in response to the instructions below. Subsequently, compare your response to the graded essays that follow.

WRITING TASK A

Consider the following comments and develop a piece of writing in response to one or more of them.

Your writing will be judged on the quality of your response to the theme; how well you organise and present your point of view, and how effectively you express yourself. You will not be judged on the views or attitudes you express.

* * * * * *

"Laws made by common consent must not be trampled on by individuals."

George Washington

"The final test of civilisation of a people is the respect they have for law."

Lewis F. Korns

"In matters of conscience, the law of the majority has no place."

Mahatma Gandhi

"In Republics, the great danger is that the majority may not sufficiently respect the rights of the minority."

James Madison

"All, too, will bear in mind this sacred principle, that though the will of the majority is in all cases to prevail, that will to be rightful must be reasonable; that the minority possess their equal rights, which equal law must protect, and to violate would be oppression."

Thomas Jefferson

SAMPLE ESSAY #1

A A A A A

The law of the majority Unimportant?

"In matters of concience the law of the majority has no place". For instance, a hs student, greatly feels peer pressure would choose not to smoke eventhough the majority of his peers feel that it is a desirable thing to do. According to the statement this student should make his choice based on what he believes not to be right, regardless of the general consesnus of his peers.

There are some situations in which the law of majority is important in matters of conscience. For instance, a politician that believes in firearms can not make a law to force his constituents to carry guns, if they are horrible opposed to such weapons in the first place. Therefore the politician, in doing what he feels is right wouldn't be able to ignore the general consensus of the people of his province about firearms because his decision about such a law would affect them as well as him.

Certain circumstances would govern whether the law of majority is important or not in matters of conscience. If a person acts in such a way that he can live with, and it doesn't have adverse effects on other people who may

IF YOU NEED MORE SPACE, CONTINUE ON THE NEXT PAGE.

A A A A A

feel quite differently, then the law of majority is unimportant. If a person's conscience tells them to act in ways that hurt others, then the conscience of the majority must be taken into account. For instance, a Christian school teacher can't force her class that is majority Jewish to sing christmas songs because she believes it's the proper thing to do during the christmas holidays. That would antagonize the class, which would have been taken into consideration when she wanted to do what's right.

IF YOU NEED MORE SPACE, CONTINUE ON THE BACK OF THIS PAGE.

Analysis of Sample Essay #1

Score
2/6 44–50

Task 1 – not really achieved. Although the statement was used in the first sentence, it was never really defined as a thesis nor otherwise defined. Encountering the typographical error "concience" instead of "conscience" or the mistake in spelling the quote in the beginning, seriously hurts the credibility of the writer. Peer evaluation or pressure is somewhat analogous to the making of laws by the majority, but quite loose as an association. For these reasons, clarity of thought and concrete examples to support a given thesis seem cloudy and unfocussed.

Task 2 – an antithesis is never really developed to the extent needed. While the politician example whom is juxtaposed in relation to a general consensus, could be developed, the idea of "forcing" people to carry weapons, seems an example, a bit absurd and reaching. The credibility of the writer is also questioned, when the use of "horrible" instead of the correct "horribly" (Para. 2, Line 2) is used adding to a general tone of inconsistency in care of grammar, and overall approach to the subject.

Task 3 – Because neither of the above tasks were completed with the necessary organisational and supportive devices and materials, providing a synthesis of arguments presented is impossible. A touchy feely context-based qualification in the surmounting to a "well, it all depends on the circumstance," is an intellectual and academic cop-out. The example of the Christian school teacher with Jewish students not forcing them to sing Christian songs, could be developed in more detail, if such an example is chosen.

Overall – some good ideas, but unfocussed, not organised to the extent needed. There seems to be some misunderstanding of the quote. The writer needs to reveal the Gandhi meaning that non-violent resistance to certain political repressions was not only necessary, but morally correct and in opposition to the laws of the majority. Hypothetical examples could be explored also: suppose that there was a law passed that said you could not protest or peaceably assemble to protest, or a law prohibiting you from enjoying "life, liberty, and the pursuit of happiness." In many ways, the subject of the essay concerns "personal liberty" vs. "collective responsibility" or "subjective reactions" to "legislative mandates or laws." This juxtaposition, or fulcrum needs to be explored and balanced to a larger degree.

Technical errors, spelling, and typographical errors deflated the essay – as previously noted. A stronger organisational pattern is needed, which follows a sequential and logical progression.

Evaluation (*see* WC 4.5): 2/6. This essay completely fails to address adequately one or more of the tasks. There may be recurring mechanical errors (i.e. spelling and grammar). Problems with analysis and organisation are typical (though organisation was fine in this instance).

> ***2*** These essays may show some problems with clarity or complexity of thought. The treatment of the writing assignment may show problems with integration or coherence. Major ideas may be underdeveloped. There may be numerous errors in mechanics, usage, or sentence structure.

A A A A A

My Rights Begin Where Yours End

In our democratic society, we have created many laws or rules gained through legislation. These rules are discussed, developed and enacted by elected officials who represent the ~~(most)~~ majority of their constituents. However, the laws produced in this manner may be in conflict with a particular individual's beliefs or values. Thus the statement suggests that when such a conflict is evident, the individuals beliefs superceed the law, rendering the rules of the majority irrelevant. "In matters of conscience, the law of the majority has no place." spoken by a man of peace regarding a non violent struggle. However, there are those who have used such ideas for darker purposes...

For example, in 1996 many churches frequented by the African-American community were set ablaze by individuals - some of whom were members of racist movements. Both arson and such race-based acts are illegal in America. As in this case, the individuals who acted in defiance of the law of majority claimed they were abiding by their own beliefs and values. Thus they acted with a clear conscience destroying the lives and communities of innocent victims. Such a crime is immoral, unacceptable and - according to the rules of

IF YOU NEED MORE SPACE, CONTINUE ON THE NEXT PAGE.

SAMPLE ESSAY #2

A A A A A

the majority – illegal. Clearly, the law of majority must supercede the conscience of the perpetrators of such a crime.

The dividing line becomes clear. Life, liberty and the pursuit of happiness are the foundations of Constitution. The concept is both logical and moral. Our conscience should be our guide as we excercise our our freedom. However, since our neighbors and fellow Americans share the same rights, someone's conscience should never be used as a reason why someone's Constitutionally protected rights are stripped away. In conclusion, one's conscience should be one's guide but when it interferes with the rights of others, the law of majority becomes more important.

IF YOU NEED MORE SPACE, CONTINUE ON THE NEXT PAGE.

Analysis of Sample Essay #2

Score
5/6 65–71

Task 1 – A quick example could help buttress Task 1 in outlining the thesis matter, where subjective liberties are at odds with social, legislative, or governmental mandates. As noted in Essay #1, hypothetical examples could be used in supporting the thesis outline. Identifying the source of the quote as Gandhi, as a man of peace, helps further establish the credibility as a writer.

Task 2 – effective transition into an antithetical notion of when a sinister turn is taken between the dialectic of individual rights-beliefs and governmental mandates. Very good *specific* example and portrayal of the paradoxes of such a balance.

Task 3 – follows a logical progression, sequential with good analysis and reasoning. Good use of quotes in relation to a most relevant document concerning this juxtaposition: The Constitution (naturally, there are many effective international, national or regional examples depending on where you live or where you attend school).

Overall – good logical sequence, completion of tasks to an above average extent, clarity of focus, good development of ideas, clear and simple style of language.

The title did not necessarily - nor correctly - represent the outline of the ideas presented to the adequacy needed. The title is somewhat ambiguous and polysemantic, having several ways to interpret. Another minor observation – rules and laws are conflated to some extent, they could be differentiated more effectively, or simply omit the use of the word "rules".

Examples of some minor technical and typographical errors – "gained" in Paragraph (P) 1, Line (L) 2 is redundant, omit; P1, L9 – "supercede" not "superceed"; P3, L2 – insert "the" before "Constitution"; P3, L3 should be "These concepts are . . ."; P3, L4 doubled "our our"; P3, L9 – "constitutionally" – use lower case.

Evaluation (*see* WC 4.5): 5/6: All tasks are addressed by this essay. The treatment of the subject is substantial but not as thorough as for a 6 point essay. While some depth, structure and good vocabulary and sentence control are exhibited, this is at a lower level than for a 6 point essay.

> ***5*** These essays show clarity of thought, with some depth or complexity. The treatment of the rhetorical assignment is generally focussed and coherent. Major ideas are well developed. A strong control of language is evident.

4.9 Frequently Asked Questions

Over the last 12 years, our Gold Standard GAMSAT Essay-correction Service has corrected thousands of student essays en route to improved GAMSAT Written Communication scores. From our experience, students tend to have similar concerns about essay writing for the GAMSAT.

How many quotes should I choose?

Your true focus should be the process of brainstorming at the start of the GS "Five-minute, Five-step Plan" (WC 4.2.8): Keeping the overall theme in mind, which quote or quotes generate(s) the best ideas?

There are students who have obtained exceptionally high scores exploring only 1 quote for their essay as there have been students who have explored 3 or more quotes. As long as you stick to the theme, the number of quotes that you choose should not be your focus. Compelling ideas which are well-illustrated must be the focus of your essay.

From our experience, an average science student without essay-writing experience tends to optimise their score by choosing 2 quotes in opposition for the argumentative essay (Writing Test A), and one quote - well explored - for the reflective essay (Writing Test B). Your personal experience and skills may lead you to a different path in order to optimise your score.

Ultimately, it all boils down to your experiences, writing skills and knowledge of the theme of the quotes.

Which quote should I choose?

Writing Test A: Consider the 3 tasks that we described as applied to the 4 or 5 quotes. Which generates the most clear, specific ideas? Can you mention dates with confidence? Can you mention names other than those that are sometimes provided alongside the quotes? Other specifics? Answering these questions will lead you naturally down the path to the ideal quote for you to optimise your score.

Writing Test B: Consider personal experiences/reflections to illustrate any of the quotes provided. If that truly does not work, try the reverse (i.e. an argumentative approach). Consider the social implication for that point of view. Any quote, within the context of the overall theme, that generates the best ideas, should be pursued with vigour.

How do I quote a statement that has been listed without any attribution in a writing task?

First, let's establish the academic protocol for quoting statements. Ideally, you would require the parenthetical after the quote: (Anonymous, Year). Considering that themes are given on-the-spot in the exam, it is unlikely that you will know the year, so you could just write: (Anonymous). This would be effective in an argumentative, formal essay such as in Writing Task A. For example: "Good friends are hard to find, harder to leave, and impossible to forget." (Anonymous)

On the other hand, if you are using an informal style (which is common for Writing Task B), then you could write something similar, as follows: As has been said anonymously, "Write a wise saying and your name will live forever."

It all boils down to style. As long as you treat the quote with as much respect as you would any quote, then your GAMSAT score is unlikely to be significantly affected by the style used regarding this issue.

As an aside: If it is a long quotation, it is unlikely to benefit your essay if you were to rewrite the whole statement. You can simply quote from the most powerful part of the statement or comment while providing context for the rest. Alternatively, you can just refer to the statement and then paraphrase it completely while providing an example or examples.

What do I do if I have strong argumentative ideas for Writing Test B?

Go with it! If your creative juices flow in a particular direction, you must go with the flow of ideas. The point of understanding the Gold Standard structure for Writing Tests A and B (WC 4.25 and WC 4.2.6) is that you keep in mind the objective. For example, even if you pursue an argumentative essay for Test B, consider the social implication and, most importantly, reflect on the personal meaning and related experience(s).

Accordingly, you can use a reflective or a personal narrative in response to Writing Test A. As discussed in WC 4.2.3, you may appeal to a reader's pathos in an argument. Besides, ACER does not impose any format for Written Communication. What they simply require is for you to generate a valuable response for the socio-cultural theme of Test A and the personal-social one in Test B. We've had past students who did well in Written Communication using the reflective approach for both tasks.

How personal is personal?

Your GAMSAT Writing Test B may include personal experiences that you are willing to share with, obviously, a stranger who is professional at marking essays (i.e. this is not your psychiatrist!!). In other words, this is unlikely to be the ideal venue to share experiences that you have never shared with anyone in your entire life.

On the other hand, "personal" must be sincere and must exemplify the point that you are trying to make. Being sincere and practicing your essay-writing skills optimise the chance that the reader buys into the experience that you are describing in your essay.

Examples of meaningful, personal expressions that, within context, seemed sincere: I wept, I felt, I failed, I was able to overcome my failure, I was hurt, I was the cause of his/her pain, I realised, I adapted, I was forced/compelled to reconsider, etc.

How many essays do top GAMSAT Written Communication students complete prior to the exam?

Top students complete 20-40 timed essays prior to the actual GAMSAT. Of course, students with natural charisma expressed by the pen or with a non-science background can get away with much less practice and still obtain a high Written Communication score.

How can I gauge my essay-writing progress?

We have placed our suggested scoring system in this book (WC 4.7). You can have someone that you respect (a friend, family member, high-school teacher or university professor), score some of your essays. ACER has a new automated GAMSAT Written Communication scoring service, which you can access by going to their website. Gold Standard has a personalised essay-correction service, which you can access at GAMSAT-prep.com.

Is there anything useful to revise for Written Communication the night before the exam?

Yes! Consider revising the answers you create for the Written Communication exercises in this book; the quotes, helpful words and Latin expressions from this book or from your personal notes; and revise the notes you take from your practice exam experiences and/or from your exposure to the various resources we have previously described. In the end, well-explored ideas combined with 2-3 powerful words and/or expressions can produce tremendous results for GAMSAT Written Communication.

What is the ideal length of a GAMSAT essay?

Unless you can think fast and type fast at the same time, you really have time for only one and a half up to two pages. The most important thing is to finish a well-organised essay with great ideas that is also easy to understand.

What level of English skills would be required in Written Communication?

Part of the assessment is being able to put your ideas and emotions in words that are clear, appropriate and accurate. This means that your spelling skills must be decent enough that you can tell the difference between "eel" and "ill" or "peach" and "pitch," for example.

You must also be able to construct complete sentences. Keep in mind that spoken English and written English have their own nuances. Colloquial terms and tone are highly discouraged. After all, you are applying for a graduate medicine program. It is only reasonable that you are expected to write formal, academic essays.

Another option is to enroll in a short-term writing class. You can inquire from your university's Student Services office to aid you in this area.

I have never been good at writing essays. My head goes blank every time I attempt to start writing. Do you have any suggestions?

You need to find out what could be causing the problem. Two common root causes are **exam anxiety** and **limited reading exposure**.

Sometimes, when you are too nervous trying to beat the limited time to write your essays, you end up with nothing essential - "your head goes blank." The solution is really very simple. Practice as often as you can. Just like any skills training, you have to keep practicing until you master the techniques.

If the problem is because you are always faced with unfamiliar topics and you have no idea what to talk about, you need to read as much varied materials as you can - news, blogs, even scientific articles, and so on. But because you are preparing for the GAMSAT, an exam that requires you to write short essays, you might want to choose short articles from which to emulate good writing and concise arguments.

Is a title important?

A title is not required but if something original or engaging comes to mind after having planned your essay, then it could be of benefit. Please avoid writing a title that says "Comment no. 1" or "Quote no. 2" though. Remember that the main purpose of a title is to catch a reader's interest, so make it interesting, witty and beautifully worded (for example, an expression from your national anthem or a Latin expression).

How much time do I need to prepare for Written Communication?

We generally suggest studying 3-6 hours per day for 3-6 months but that includes successful preparation for all 3 GAMSAT sections. Of course, the caveat being that those are averages; due to a wide range of life experiences, some candidates will need much more time while others may only need 1-2 weeks of preparation to obtain a GAMSAT score sufficient for admissions.

Developing language skills, and a writing style that suits you best, can indeed take some time: weeks or months for most, years for some (clearly, we are discussing GAMSAT success and not the Pulitzer Prize). The key is to determine your strengths and weaknesses months before the exam and then practice, practice, practice.

4.10 Common Grammatical Errors

Please do not read the following section unless either it is more than 6 weeks before the real exam or you have done some practice essays and you find that generating ideas and producing a well-structured essay is no longer challenging. At this point, improving details such as grammar and flexibility in the use of language can now become more interesting to explore as you aim to go from a very good score to an excellent score.

Some Basic Concepts

By definition, a sentence has the following properties:

it contains a *subject*

it contains a *verb*

it expresses a *complete thought*

E.g., the sentence *"China prospers."* has a subject: "China"; a verb: "prospers"; and it conveys a complete thought or idea that makes sense.

Most sentences also have an *object* (receiver of the action); e.g., in the sentence "Mary baked a cake," the object is "a cake."

Run-on Sentences (fused sentences)

Incorrect usage	Correct usage	Explanation
He watched the movie ten times he really loved it.	He watched the movie ten times. He really loved it. He watched the movie ten times; he really loved it. He watched the movie ten times, for he really loved it. Since he really loved the movie, he watched it ten times.	Run-on sentences occur when two main clauses have no punctuation between them. Separate the two main ideas into separate complete sentences and punctuate each properly. Use a conjunction preceded by a comma to combine two ideas. Subordinate one of the main ideas into a clause.

Comma Faults (comma splices)

Incorrect usage	Correct usage	Explanations
He watched the movie ten times, he really loved it.	He watched the movie ten times, for he really loved it. He watched the movie ten times; he really loved it.	Comma faults occur when two main clauses are joined by only a comma. Use comma before a conjunction (*and, but, for, nor, or, so,* or *yet*) to join two complete thoughts (sentences). Use a semicolon to join two sentences. Omit the use of a conjunction, and start the second sentence in lowercase. Form two complete thoughts as separate sentences with the proper end marks. (*See* preceding example.) Join two thoughts by subordinating one of them. (*See* preceding example.)

Sentence Fragments

Incorrect usage	Correct usage	Explanation
Luke can read a book. And memorise it right after.	Luke can read a book and memorise it right after.	A sentence must have a subject and a verb.

Faulty Subordination

Incorrect usage	Correct usage	Explanation
I gazed out of the bus window, noticing a person getting mugged.	Gazing out of the bus window, I noticed a person getting mugged.	Place what you want to emphasise in the main clause, not the subordinate clause. Here the mugging should be emphasised and so should be in the main clause.

Errors in Subject-Verb Agreement

Rule: The verb should agree with the subject in terms of number (singular or plural) and person (first, second, or third).

Incorrect usage	Correct usage	Explanation
There is no glasses.	There are no glasses.	In this sentence, the subject is *glasses*, not there. *glasses* is plural; therefore, the verb should be plural (i.e. *are*).
She like diamonds.	She likes diamonds.	The subject *she* is in the second person, and is singular; therefore, the verb should also be in the second person, and be singular (i.e. *likes*).
Neither Emma nor Harry were there.	Neither Emma nor Harry was there.	In sentences where subjects are joined by *or* or *nor*, the verb agrees with the subject closer to it. In this example, "Harry" is the nearer subject. It is singular, so the verb should be also.
Neither Mary nor the others was there.	Neither Mary nor the others were there.	"Others" is the subject that is nearer to the verb. It is plural, so the verb should be also.
All of the team were there.	All of the team was there.	"Team" is singular, so the verb should be also.
All the players was present.	All the players were present.	"Players" is plural, so the verb should be also.
There are a variety of fruits.	There is a variety of fruits.	"Variety" is singular.
	There is a lot of birds here *or* there are a lot of birds here.	Both are correct. The first is correct since "lot" is singular. The second is correct because it is gaining acceptance through popular use.
Here is your shoes and tie.	Here are shoes and tie.	This sentence is in the inverted order, i.e., the subject/s come/s after the verb. When re-stated in the normal order, this sentence will be: *Your shoes and tie are here.* Subjects joined by *and* always take the plural form. Therefore, "shoes and tie" is plural, so the verb should be also.

Incorrect usage	Correct usage	Explanation
Fiona is one of the worst singers who has performed in this bar.	Fiona is one of the worst singers who have performed in this bar.	When relative pronouns *who*, *which*, or *that* are used as subjects of dependent adjective clauses, the verb of the adjective clause must agree in number with the antecedent of the pronoun. In this sentence, the antecedent of *who* is *singers*. "Singers" is plural, so the verb should be also (i.e. "have").
"I forget" or "I forgot".	I've forgotten.	Note that "I often forget" and "I forgot my umbrella yesterday" are correct.
Everybody are happy with the results.	Everybody is happy with the results.	Words like *everybody, everyone, everything, somebody, someone, each, either, nothing* and *anything* are examples of indefinite pronouns in singular form. Always remember that only the following are indefinite pronouns that are plural in form: *both, few, many, others,* and *several*. *All, any, more, most, none, some* may take singular or plural forms depending on the context of the sentence.
The queen, together with invited guests, face the media.	The queen, together with invited guests, faces the media.	The subject in this sentence is "queen". "Invited guests" is a noun of the intervening phrase that merely adds information about the subject. "Queen" is singular, so the verb should be also in its singular form, "faces".
Two-thirds of the project were assigned to me.	Two-thirds of the project was assigned to me.	When the subject is a fraction, the verb agrees with the noun in the of-phrase (i.e. "project").
The number of applicants remain unaccounted.	The number of applicants remains unaccounted.	*The number of* is always singular. *A number of* is always plural.

Errors in Noun-Pronoun Agreement

Rule: Pronouns should agree with their nouns in terms of number (singular or plural), person (first, second, or third), and gender (masculine or feminine).

Incorrect usage	Correct usage	Explanation
Did everyone remember their assignment?	Did everyone remember his assignment?	*Everyone* is singular, so the pronoun should be as well.
It was them who apologised.	It was they who apologised.	The nominative case (I, you, he, she, it, we, you, they, who) is used following some form of the verb *to be*.
If I were him, I would go.	If I were he, I would go.	As above.
It is me.	It is I.	As above.
Whom will succeed?	Who will succeed?	A simple rule-of-thumb is to use "who" when "he" would also make sense; and use "whom" when "him" would also make sense (e.g. "Him will succeed" does not sound right, while "he will succeed" does).
Who did you give it to?	Whom did you give it to?	As above. "You gave it to he" does not sound right, while "you gave it to him" does. Thus, use "whom".
It belongs to he and I.	It belongs to him and me.	The *objective* case of pronoun (i.e. me, you, him, her, it, us, you, them, whom) is used as the object of a preposition, such as "to".
Hugh fired he.	Hugh hired him.	The *objective* case of pronoun (i.e. me, you, him, her, it, us, you, them, whom) is used as the *object* of a verb.
He is as proficient as me.	He is as proficient as I.	Try stretching the sentence out: "He is as proficient as *I am proficient*, not "he is as proficient as *me am proficient*."
He was in the same class as us.	He was in the same class as we.	Try stretching the sentence out: "He was in the same class as *we were in*."
I trust Bob more than he.	I trust Bob more than him.	Try stretching the sentence out: "I trust Bob more than *I trust him*."
Now sing without me coaching you.	Now sing without my coaching you.	Use the *possessive* case of the pronoun (i.e. my, your, his, her, its, our, your, their, whose) in sentences like this.

Special Problems in Pronoun Agreement

Incorrect usage	Correct usage	Explanation
The movie was disappointing because *they* never made the plot seem realistic.	The *movie* was disappointing because *it* never made the plot seem realistic. The movie was disappointing because *the writers* never made the plot seem realistic.	Pronoun must agree with antecedents that are either clearly stated or understood. Otherwise, use a specific noun.
In 17th century England, *you* had to choose between following the Church or the King.	In 17th century England, *Puritans* had to choose between following the Church or the King.	Use *YOU* only when the reference is truly addressed to the reader.
Charles asked *William* about the state of his marriage. William tried to evade the topic, but confused about the situation, *he* tried to carry on a pleasant conversation.	*Charles* asked *William* about the state of his marriage. *William* tried to evade the topic, but confused about the situation, *Charles* tried to carry on a pleasant conversation.	Always use a pronoun close enough to its antecedent to avoid confusion.
I placed my passport in my bag, but I can't find *it*.	I placed my passport in my bag, but I can't find *my bag*.	Use pronouns to refer to an obvious antecedent.

Dangling Modifiers

Rule: Avoid dangling modifiers (i.e. adjectives or adverbs that do not refer to the noun or pronoun they are intended to refer to).

Incorrect usage	Correct usage	Explanation
While dialling the phone, the lights went out.	While *I was* dialling the phone, the lights went out.	The modifying phrase "while dialling the phone" does not refer to a particular noun or pronoun (i.e. it dangles).
After attending the mass, pizza was eaten.	After attending the mass, we ate pizza.	As above.

Misplaced Modifiers

Incorrect usage	Correct usage	Explanation
Nina won almost 1 million euros.	Nina almost won 1 million euros.	The first sentence does not mean what it is intended to mean. The modifier "almost" is misplaced.
I only want you.	I want only you.	Same as above.

"Were" **to be used in the Subjunctive Mood**

Rule: Use *"were"* in the subjunctive mood, i.e. when expressing a wish, regret, or a condition that does not exist.

Incorrect usage	Correct usage	Explanation
If I was prettier, I would be famous.	If I were prettier, I would be famous.	This sentence is in the subjunctive mood.
Mum treats him as if he is a slave.	Mum treats him as if he were a slave.	As above.

That, Which, and Who

Incorrect usage	Correct usage	Explanation
This is the novel which he loved.	This is the novel that he loved.	When commas are not used, use "that".
This gown, that is designed by Monique, is expensive and elegant.	This gown, which is designed by Monique, is expensive and elegant.	When commas are used, use "which".
She is the person that designed the gown.	She is the person who designed the gown.	For persons, use "who". Do not use "who" for animals.
The President, which is an avid golfer, was on the course.	The President, who is an avid golfer, was on the course.	For persons, use "who", even when commas are used.

Note: Often the above pronouns can be omitted making a sentence more concise. Thus:

This is the novel he loved. ("That" is implied.) This gown, designed by Monique, is expensive and elegant. She designed the gown. The President, an avid golfer, was on the course.

Faulty Parallelism

Incorrect usage	Correct usage	Explanation
She likes to read, swim and shopping a lot.	She likes to read, swim and shop a lot. She likes to read, to swim and to shop a lot.	Similar ideas should be expressed in grammatically similar forms. (e.g., nouns with nouns, adjectives with adjectives, words with words, phrases with phrases)
The professor was asked to submit his report quick and accurately.	The professor was asked to submit his report quickly and accurately.	Similar ideas should be expressed in grammatically similar structures (i.e. same word order, consistent verb tenses).

Mixed Constructions

Incorrect usage	Correct usage	Explanation
Will asked Lizzie to marry him?	Will asked Lizzie to marry him?	Don't mix a statement with a question.
The reason is because I don't have a nanny.	The reason is that I don't have a nanny.	Don't mix two different sentence constructions.

Split Infinitives

Incorrect usage	Correct usage	Explanation
I need to mentally prepare.	I need to prepare mentally.	"To prepare" is an infinitive. Splitting infinitives with other words tends to be awkward.

Commas

Incorrect usage	Correct usage	Explanation
Uncle has money, wealth and power.	Uncle has money, wealth, and power.	Use a comma before the last item in a series to avoid any confusion.
The food was served late cold and smelly.	The food was served late, cold, and smelly.	Use commas to separate adjectives that could be joined with "and." You could say that "the food was served late and cold and smelly."
Jonas is a popular, varsity player.	Jonas is a popular varsity player.	Don't use commas to separate adjectives that could not be joined with "and." It would be ridiculous to say that " Jonas is a popular and varsity player."

Incorrect usage	Correct usage	Explanation
You wait here, and I'll get your coat.	You wait here and I'll get your coat.	Don't use a comma to set off clauses that are short or have the same subject. However, always use a comma before "for", "so," and "yet" to avoid confusion.
The doctor gave detailed precise instructions to the nurse.	The doctor gave detailed, precise instructions to the nurse.	Use commas to separate adjectives of same or equal rank.
India has a rigid, social caste system.	India has a rigid social caste system.	Do not use commas to separate adjectives that must stay in a specific order.

Semicolons

Incorrect usage	Correct usage	Explanation
The car is old, however, it is in good condition.	The car is old; however, it is in good condition. The car is old; it is, however, in good condition.	Use a semicolon with a conjunctive adverb (e.g. nevertheless, however, otherwise, consequently, thus, therefore, meanwhile, moreover, furthermore).

Apostrophes

Correct usage	Explanation
Maggie Holmes' dog is lost. Maggie Holmes 's dog is lost.	Since there is disagreement on which is correct, both are acceptable.
The girl's doll fell in the mud. The girls' doll fell in the mud.	Common errors arise when apostrophes are misplaced in singular and plural nouns. In the first sentence, placing the apostrophe in between the noun and an *s* indicates a singular noun. In the second sentence, an apostrophe placed after a plural noun hints that the "doll" is commonly owned by at least two girls.

Troublesome Verbs

TRANSITIVE (followed by an object)	**INTRANSITIVE** (not followed by an object)
raise, raising, raised: The farmer is raising chickens.	**rise, rising, rose**: The moon is rising.
lay, laying, laid: I am laying the dress on the bed.	**lie, lying, lain**: I am lying on the bed.

"A" **or** *"The"*

Correct usage	Explanation
I dated **the** cheerleader back in college.	The definite article **the** is used when referring to a specific subject or member of a group. The speaker in the sentence could have been acquainted with many cheerleaders; but he was able to date only one particular cheerleader.
I dated **a** cheerleader back in college.	Use the indefinite article **a** to refer to a non-specific subject. The sentence implies that the speaker dated someone who could have been any member of a cheerleading group.

Proper Usage of *"The"*

• The Thames flow through Oxford and London. • The Gibson Desert is home to indigenous Australians. • Myths say that Santa Claus lives in the North Pole. • The equator is approximately 3,500 miles from the southernmost part of the United Kingdom. • The Chinese are hardworking people.	USE **the** when referring to • the proper names of rivers, oceans and seas; • deserts, forests, gulfs, and peninsulas • geographical areas • points on the globe • some countries like *the* Netherlands, *the* Dominican Republic, *the* Philippines, *the* United States • the people of a nation
Anna shops in Bond Street. Blue Lake attracts many tourists in Australia. St. Patrick's Island is a sanctuary for seabirds. Galtymore ranks 14th among Ireland's highest mountain peak. English is the main language used in the United Kingdom.	DO NOT USE **the** when referring to • street names • names of lakes except with a group of lakes • bays • most countries/territories but NOT cities, states or towns • names of mountains in general • names of continents • names of islands except with island chains • names of languages and nationalities

Verb or Participle

Not all verbs demonstrate an action. There are those that merely express a condition or an existence. These are called linking verbs. Words that describe (adjectives) or identify (another noun) should follow the linking verb.

Examples:

Incorrect Usage	Correct Usage
Nicole Kidman **sounds** sarcastically in the interview.	Nicole Kidman **sounds** sarcastic in the interview. The verb "sounds" expresses the state of emotions (sarcastic) of the subject (Nicole Kidman) at the time of the interview.
	Sir Edward Hallstrom **is** a philanthropist. The verb "is" connects the noun "philanthropist" to the subject "Sir Edward Hallstrom".

Participles are words that look like verbs but function in the sentence as nouns.

Example: **Exploring** Lake Argyle is one of the most wonderful outdoor adventures in Australia.
"Exploring" is a participle that functions as the noun-subject in the sentence and should not be confused with the main verb "is".

Common errors involving confusion between verbs and participles lead to **Sentence Fragments.**

Incorrect Usage	Correct Usage	Explanation
Dancing on her toes. The ballerina **was** superb.	**Dancing** on her toes, the ballerina **was** superb.	The main thought of the sentence is a description of the level of performance of the subject (ballerina) - "superb". The action word "dancing" merely adds information about what the subject (ballerina) does.

4.11 Written Communication Practice Worksheets

Written Communication Practice Worksheet I (Formulating the Thesis Statement)

Comment #	Repeated words	Ideas for or against the subject
1		
2		
3		
4		
5		
Topic:		
Theme or Issue:		
My Debatable Claim		

Written Communication Practice Worksheet II (Writing the Introduction)

This is where you express your interpretation of the comments' theme. You may state it as a direct statement or you may use a creative device.	
This is where you expound your ideas in relation to your initial statement by quoting or paraphrasing one or two of the given comments. Alternatively, you can continue discussing your narrative or metaphor.	
Your last sentence in the paragraph is your thesis statement. Make sure that it is clear, and it is debatable claim.	

Written Communication Practice Worksheet III (Task A Template)
Note: This template may also be used if you are more comfortable using an argumentative format for Writing Task B.

(Optional) Choose a title that summarises - in one short phrase - the overall idea of your essay.	
This is your introductory paragraph. Remember to include the following: - Aim to open with a catchy statement or anecdote - Express what the overall theme or one of the comments means to you - Include your debatable thesis statement in the last sentence of the paragraph (**Note:** Sometimes, if your introduction is too lengthy, you can discuss your thesis statement in the second paragraph.)	
In this paragraph, your aim is to explain and support your thesis statement. - Give one reason or argument in support of your thesis - Provide a concrete example or examples to support your argument - Explain how the examples relate to the argument	

This is where you present the strongest counterargument to your thesis. - Your counterargument should be related or parallel to the thesis' supporting example - Provide a clear illustration of your counter-argument's example.	
This is the paragraph where you show that your thesis' arguments are superior to the antithesis. Your aim here is to show that you have carefully considered all arguments for and against your idea and you have made up your mind to choose your arguments because it is better than the best opposition to it.	
This is your closing paragraph. - Summarise the main ideas discussed in the preceding paragraphs. - Tie up or reconcile conflicting ideas. - Propose your plan of action for the consideration of the reader - End with a memorable statement.	

Written Communication Practice Worksheet IV (Task B Template)

Note: This template may also be used if you are more comfortable using a personal piece for Writing Task A.

(Optional) Choose a title that summarises - in one short phrase - the overall idea of your essay.	
This is your introductory paragraph. Remember to explain: - what the comment's mean to you. - why you agree or disagree with the comment's idea. Briefly present your thesis statement towards the end of the paragraph.	
This is where you begin your personal narrative. It must be about an event that is pivotal in your life. It must also be relevant to the theme of the comments and/or your thesis.	

This is where you share your realisations from the personal narrative. Describe: - how you felt - how you thought and - what made you change your mind or point of view **There must be a 'before-and-after' description of your state of mind and state of heart.**	
This is where you state an application of your personal realisation. Cite a social problem that is relevant to your experience. How can your life-lesson serve as an inspiration to those who may be similarly situated? What new perspectives can you offer to the social problem that you cited?	

4.12 Breaking the Rules: Exploring Creativity

Now that you have understood the basic requirements and criteria for each writing task, you can start exploring creative ways of presenting your ideas without necessarily following the 'rules' to a tee. If you have an excellent command of the English language and believe that you have what it takes to come up with outstanding, unique Written Communication pieces on exam day, then you may consider adopting the following options for 'breaking the rules'. The key is to practice and refine your format, making sure that you demonstrate sophisticated writing and thinking skills.

- Analogy

You can use an object as a point of reference to express your views and feelings on a theme. For example, if you are into photography or filmmaking as a hobby, you could describe different stages of your argument as "scenes" that build up to a conclusion or a personal realisation. *See* WC 4.2.2 for more examples of analogy, metaphor, and simile.

- Letter

Even in Writing Task A, you can choose to write a "Letter to the Editor" or a "Dear Madam Prime Minister / Mr President" letter to express your strong opinion on an important sociocultural issue. Your letter must still be evidence-based but the letter format and tone will make your piece quite interesting for the markers to read.

For the more personal Writing Task B, you can write a "Dear Mum" or "Dear Dad" letter. A break-up letter or a resignation letter would also be unique when discussing a personal issue (whether it is fictional or not) that most readers would find relatable.

- Short Story

You can write a fictional short story, a fairy tale or a historical narrative. Depending on your academic background and training, writing in this format can take several practice in order to generate an engaging story which is highly relevant to the given theme, the appropriate narrative tone, relatable characters, etc.

- Debate or Conversation

You can also write a hypothetical debate between two of the authors who are quoted in the list of comments.

- Poem
- Diary Entry
- Social Media Post

You will find many creative touches, as well as strong conventional approaches to writing essays, in the next section (WC 5.1).

5.1 Gold Ideas

One of the main ingredients in obtaining an excellent Written Communication score is constant practice. Write as many essays as you can based on as many themes that you can reasonably explore during your GAMSAT preparation timetable (*see* the table of themes from past exams in WC 4.1). You will note that many of the real past Written Communication topics can be prescribed a more broad categorisation. For example, affirmative action and meritocracy fall under the general topic of equality; optimism, humour, and life goals are quite germane to the theme of happiness, and so forth.

This means that you can actually prepare and polish possible arguments, stories, and supporting examples which you can conveniently use in case you encounter a related theme in the writing tasks during your exam. Most importantly, train your mind to form opinions on important social, cultural and personal issues, which you can support with sound and concrete evidence.

The following essays are meant to expose you to various perspectives on typical Written Communication topics, as well as different presentation styles. These essays were submitted to our GS Essay-correction Service by actual students under timed conditions, hence you may observe some grammatical errors - albeit minimal and tolerable - in some of the pieces. These written responses will hopefully advance your development of unique and creative ideas to help you produce punchy Written Communication essays that offer fresh insights vis-à-vis the themes presented to you on exam day. And finally, consider taking very brief notes ('Gold Notes', at most 2-3 sentences per essay) especially when you encounter content that impresses you in some way. Enjoy!

Please note: Your essay responses for Written Communication, for the real GAMSAT, will undergo an online plagiarism investigation. This includes third-party sources of content, as well as a plagiarism verification against ACER's GAMSAT database of previously submitted responses. Needless to say, ACER views plagiarism as an unacceptable act of misconduct. Do not try to memorise an essay. Discover your inner creative self, and then practice, practice, practice.

Also note that there are 40 Task A model essays and 40 Task B model essays in this book, with another 20⁺ model essays in your gamsat-prep.com account.

5.1.1 Writing Task A Model Essays

Comment Set A

Comment 1

Technology makes it possible for people to gain control over everything, except over technology.

****

Comment 2

Humanity is acquiring all the right technology for all the wrong reasons.

****

Comment 3

If it keeps up, man will atrophy all his limbs but the push-button finger.

****

Comment 4

The real danger is not that computers will begin to think like men, but that men will begin to think like computers.

****

Comment 5

It has become appallingly obvious that our technology has exceeded our humanity.

Task A: Essay Sample 1
Comment Set A

The Chinese philosopher Laotse once said that all that was essential was in the vacuum. The usefulness of a jug, he claimed, was in the empty space to hold water. Like Laotse's jug, the human mind thrives on wandering freely. Ironically it is this very capacity to think freely that has constructed a system which inhibits our freedom. Although technology improves our lives in numerous profound ways, it is also a dangerous, uncontrollable vice that threatens the nature of human existence.

It would be impossible to deny the positive effects of technology in our world. With tools, man conquered his fear of animals. With agriculture, his fear of starvation too withered. Since the industrial revolution, unprecedented advancements in technology have resulted in a standard of living simply unimaginable to our ancestors who went before us.

Every innovation as a single development seems like a simple step towards a more convenient life. However it is difficult to see the pernicious effects of these seemingly innocuous developments as a whole. Technological pleasures enjoyed responsibly can have huge benefits in our lives, but these days many of us are addicted to technology to the extent that we are constantly seeking passive entertainment and the very nature of human interaction is being morphed in a scary way.

As all activities become cheaper our reliance on each other for help dwindles. It's an easily observable fact that people tend to keep to themselves more now than they did, say, 30 years ago. Another painful irony is that of mobile communication. Messaging apps like facebook claim to connect us with people all over the world, but this type of communication is no substitute for talking face to face. However, it does reduce the amount of time people spend out meeting each other. We see this particularly in younger kids. Their idea of communication is very distorted in comparison with what we know, and not in a positive way. These screens are a screen that protects us from embarrassing interactions and difficult experience.

Facing up to difficult experiences, rather than letting them fester in the woods of denial, is the bedrock of clinical psychology. These inconveniences, that technology tries to eradicate, are hard-wired into our brains. When we choose to ignore them with the veil of comfort we fail to treat them or better understand ourselves.

To conclude, undoubtedly the benefits of technology are abundant. However the problems modern technology addresses are often innate characteristics of being human that are better off confronted than simply avoided. It is important that we try to acknowledge the dangers of technology so that we can be wary of the road down which they take us, and so that it remains a tool for us, not the other way around.

Task A: Essay Sample 2
Comment Set A

Níl Saol gan Locht

One of the biggest challenges of our generation is the misuse of technology. Technology originally was invented to make life 'easier'. It has brought about countless problems with detrimental consequences. It can be seen as both good and bad depending on which area you look at, for example in healthcare it is revolutionary but with regards to its impact on mental health, it is egregious. Some people believe technology benefits society, in contrast, others are of the opinion we would be better off without it. The ubiquitous question is - does technology improve or damage society?

Technology, when used correctly has had an amazing impact on society. According to The Economist, it's use in diagnostic machinery in healthcare has decreased deaths from heart disease by half since 1980. It is an immense aid in statistics, allowing us to assess covid-19 reproduction, identify key outbreak zones and communicate safety measures to the public. It allows family members and friends to keep in contact, some who may have not seen each other for years due to geographical distances etc, some people have even found long lost family members online!

However, there is no doubt that it is a hindrance on society, we have little tolerance for others, are less conversational and less empathetic. We are often completely unaware of our surroundings as we are hiding behind little screens, in a different world altogether. It has a detrimental impact on mental health. According to 'The Social Dilemma' plastic surgeons are seeing a huge amount of young, impressionable people wanting amendments made to their faces for the 'filter effect' that is plastered over Instagram and Snapchat.

On social platforms we are being exploited, we are the product. Advertisers pay platforms such as Facebook, Twitter, Instagram to advertise products, our activity is monitored (which we agree to when setting up an account) and ads are then presented to us numerous times every minute depending on what topics, discussions or photos we pay the most attention to on the platform. In this instance technology is the puppeteer and we are merely the puppets.

Technology, without question is good but to say it is 100% beneficial would be a myopic view, it has good and bad aspects. Undeniably, it brings about more problems than it solves. Many members of society are slaves to it, it is spiralling out of control. As said by Albert Einstein, 'it has become appallingly obvious that our technology has exceeded our humanity'.

To conclude, technology is beneficial to all when used correctly. Currently, it is spiralling out of control but one thing we must remember is that mankind are the ones inventing and developing technology, we have the both the power and the responsibility to control its use. As the Irish saying goes, 'Níl saol gan locht', there is nothing without a fault.

Comment Set B

Comment 1

One can possess a different function and still be equal in essence and worth.

****

Comment 2

Before God we are all equally wise - and equally foolish.

****

Comment 3

Full equality may become possible the day we are set up like a row of identical tin soldiers.

****

Comment 4

All animals are equal, but some animals are more equal than others.

Task A: Essay Sample 3
Comment Set B

The debate of equality can be approached by comparing the idealism with the reality. Many believe that all humans beings are fundamentally the same. Others argue that this is not possible as equality does not exist within society. I believe that human equality exists inside all of us yet fails to manifest itself in society.

All of humanity is fundamentally the same. The word fundamental is used here as a blanket term encompassing the core values of that comprise human nature, such as love and fear. Just before committing to jumping out of a plane to sky-dive, everyone experiences fear. Some are crippled and others are enthralled, but it is an innate response that all humans experience. With the exception of psychopaths and sociopaths, when wired up to an electroencephalograph (EEG) in order to have cerebral data taken and analysed, all individuals have surges in certain hormones and increased activity in specific areas of the brain when exposed to photos of happy infants. In almost every culture, community and companionship are central. People need human connection to survive and thrive because fundamentally, we are all the same. It is puzzling then to consider that by no means does that fundamental similarity surge out and manifest itself as a truly equal global civilisation.

Equality does not exist. People may all be created equal, but they are certainly not treated so. Take Australia for example, where Indigenous Australians make up thirty percent of all prisoners despite comprising a meagre three percent of the population. If humans are all fundamentally equal, how is it that they can have such vastly different experiences of the world? Even dating back to the agricultural revolution there is clear evidence of hierarchies in which the majority of people would labour long hours on the farm in order to contribute to the growing wealth of a select few. This phenomenon was aptly named by Karl Marx as primitive accumulation in one of his many scathing analyses of capitalism. The exact cause of these societal divisions are unclear, however, their existence poses a compelling argument that humans are in fact not all created equal.

Human nature is consistent, society is not. Societal divisions make it clear that when people are given an opportunity to improve the quality of their lives, they will take it. There have been instances in history of black societies enslaving white people, which supports the idea that if given the opportunity we are all prone to take it. Be it greed, fear or hatred, whatever the cause for societal division is, it exists in all of us.

As demonstrated by any situation that triggers the human instinct, we are all fundamentally equal. It is the divisions that occur outside ourselves, on a societal scale, that make one doubt the truth of this assertion. This doubt is quelled by the explanation that it is in fact human nature to take opportunities that will increase the chances of one's own survival, and is merely circumstance that determines who gets to take that opportunity. Humans are fundamentally equal, society is not.

Task A: Essay Sample 4
Comment Set B

Apocryphal equality in the modern society

Racism, nationalism, sexism - these are all doctrines directly contradicting social equality of the modern society. A myopic view may argue the discrimination based on socio-economical, racial, or sexuality has improved in the modern society like never before. However, the recent events suggest retro-progressing equality, as well as new sources of discrimination presented by the complex milieu of the modern society.

Since the formation of the Islamic State and increasing number of terrorist attacks against Western nations, the conflict between religious groups, as well as advocate and antagonist of nationalism, is unprecedentedly tempestuous. Due to the recent atrocities committed by religious extremists, there are increasing protests regarding the view of nationalism, and to some extremities, neo-Nazism. These ideologies that directly afflict the pursuit of social equality of mankind through centuries, are growing among the populace of victimised countries.

It is difficult to argue that in the last millennium, the equality of the mankind was continuously ameliorated through various efforts. The prohibition of slavery, approval of female election rights, collapse of caste system are just a few representations of persistent pursuit for social equality. Specifically, in the last decade, there is also an increasing effort to address the issues of inequalities, including feminism, same-sex marriage, or campaigns against racism. It is undeniable that the mankind has indeed made a significant progress and these are just a few evidences that represent pursuit of equality for all.

Unfortunately, these attempts, not to dismiss the virtuous intentions, have presented new problems against equality. In pursuit for sexual equality, or feminism, some governments have proposed the idea of quotas for female employers for a given job. Though implemented in positive ideology, this paradigm was resulted in reverse discrimination of the male workers, which has to pass significantly more fierce competition. This means that if a male and a female worker are equally potent and capable, one is more likely to get the job than the other. The virtuous intention of a policy does not necessarily result in a positive or amendment of negative phenomenon.

Communism, for example, is an ideology for the financial equality of the populace. However, it has been shown that the system does not properly operate through the examples of disintegration of Soviet Union. North Korea is the last truly communist country in the world, and the nation prevails of extreme corruption, brainwashing, and deformed distribution of wealth. Is democracy the paragon of the modern society then? The society that operates through the means of money has presented us new sources of discrimination. Those in socioeconomically disadvantaged backgrounds are unknowingly discriminated from the opportunities in terms of education and career options.

It is, therefore, impossible for the mankind to address flawless solution to address every single aspect of social inequality in terms of racial, sexual, or economical discrimination. As the quote "Full equality may become possible the day we are set up like a row of identical tin soldiers", the complex milieu of the modern society unremittingly presents new sources of discrimination and inequality. The modern society is still prevalent of inequalities sourced from traditional and newly-formed ideas, thus the governments and civilians around the globe are faced with unprecedented duty to tackle the issue.

Comment Set C

Comment 1

Nothing in Nature is random … A thing appears random only through the incompleteness of our knowledge.

****

Comment 2

God does not play dice with the universe.

****

Comment 3

The nature of the universe is fairly whimsical and nonsensical. In the most somber, beatific peacefulness there's complete chaos and maniacal laughter.

****

Comment 4

Chaos often breeds life when order breeds habit.

Task A: Essay Sample 5
Comment Set C

Is the world too perfect and well-ordered to have been created simply by chance?

We live in a universe surrounded and shaped by structure, design and complexity. When one takes the time to sit back and marvel at the spectacle of human life upon Earth, it evokes the question as to whether something so astonishing, so perfect, could really just exist due to chance. The debate as to whether the universe had a creator, some supernatural being such as a God, has long been a topic of discussion, often pitted against scientific theories surrounding the Big Bang, and the random creation of life on Earth and evolution. This essay will explore some of the major arguments within this debate, and will aim to find balance and reason in both sides of the topic.

Earth appears so far advanced, complex and diverse that the possibility of existing purely due to chance and some astronomical collision billions of years ago, is hard to get one's head around. Humans possess so much knowledge, and so much beauty in life, and Earth appears so far superior to other planets within the solar system, that the idea of a creator governing this development can seem like a more plausible and desirable explanation to its existence. The creator paves the way for life to exist, paves the way for humans to engage and interact with such superior communicative ability, and paves the way for technology to advance at such a complex and alarming rate. Proponents to the idea of a universal creator would argue that if we did have a great divine power who was responsible and had the ability to produce this 'perfect' world, then why did this creator allow for design errors leading to, for example, natural disasters. Destructive and devastating earthquakes, tsunamis and wild fires that obliterate homes and lives surely cannot be the work of a divine creator? They would argue that these occurrences are strong evidence that, while life was created by chance, it wasn't created perfect and that natural disasters are a reminder of how close humans were to never existing and how lucky we are to be able to, usually, peacefully co-exist. This line of thinking can be countered with the idea that life wouldn't be perfect or considered worthwhile unless we had negatives to help us better appreciate the positives. Natural disasters, crime and suffering are reminders from the creator that we must be thankful and appreciate the good in life. Everything serves a purpose and this suffering provides balance to world, 'Nothing in Nature is random ... A thing appears random only through the incompleteness of our knowledge'.

This debate often searches for the inadequacies or gaps lacking in each side of the arguments. Those who believe in a divine creator would argue that the theory of the Big Bang, and the creation of the universe due to an astronomical event many years prior to life on Earth, lacks any real evidence to suggest this, something that all scientific theories are grounded on. This lack of concrete evidence or proof therefore leaves the door open to speculation, and the search for a more fitting answer to why we exist, and why we exist so comfortably and so conveniently. The idea of an external creator provides comfort to these soul- searching questions. However, on the other hand, the same argument could be rebounded back to those who believe the order and design of the world wasn't by chance. What evidence is there to solidify this argument, bar sheer speculation? The religious type who believes in God as a divine being and ruler of the universe may use evidence of miracles as reason to argue its existence. The fact of the matter is, neither side can really diffuse the argument of the other, and that is why this deep debate has stood the test of time.

I believe there are strengths to both sides, but along with that, also inadequacies. I have been one to marvel at the seemingly perfect and well-ordered nature of the world we live in, and I too have questioned why Earth became so. I feel that some degree of structure must be involved in the creation of something now so complex, but where or how that came about I cannot say, but I also do not believe it was simply just a one-off random event.

Comment Set D

Comment 1

Cooperation is the thorough conviction that nobody can get there unless everybody gets there.

****

Comment 2

You will own the whole world when you no longer want to own the whole world.

****

Comment 3

It is amazing how much you can accomplish when it doesn't matter who gets the credit.

****

Comment 4

No man is an island.

Task A: Essay Sample 6
Comment Set D

In the dynamic flux of change in the world today it has never been more vital that humans cooperate. Unfortunately, world leaders are often distracted from effective governance by political squabbles. However, the best mindset for strong leadership is one which prizes teamwork, based on a conviction that "nobody can get there unless everybody gets there".

It is often when personal interests are put aside, that group cooperation is able to flourish. In the Australian response to the coronavirus pandemic, the National Cabinet has displayed a commendable model of leadership. State and Territory heads along with the Prime minister from both Labour and Liberal sides of politics have regularly worked together to coordinate public health measures. As members of the cabinet responded positively to the collaborative approach, laying aside partisanship, they demonstrated the power of cooperation to achieve results, evidenced in the successful "flattening of the curve". Although there have been moments where premiers have disagreed on the timing of measures, there has been mutual respect among cabinet members and our federal system accounts for differences between states. Thus, good communication and respect, with a common goal, can bring forth exemplary cooperation and leadership.

On the other hand, too much personal interest destroys a cooperative approach. The past decade or so of Australian politics has often been tumultuous, characterised by extreme partisanship and internal party disorder. With a number of surprising moments where the Prime Minister was ousted and a new one sworn in almost overnight, there was sense among the public that Australian politicians were becoming too self-interested. A constant reshuffling of personnel makes for an inefficient system of governance. Furthermore, the cycling through too many new prime ministers in a short period of time was seen as indulgent as retired prime ministers are supported by the public purse. Therefore, many citizens would have rather seen political parties support the leader rather than constantly undermine confidence. No doubt this would involve some compromise to personal beliefs at times. Thus cooperation requires that we put aside some of our personal differences in the interest of the efficient outcomes for the collective.

However, when ideological differences are staunch and regarded as important, cooperation is more challenging. When Australia, supported by other nations, recently led a motion for an independent inquiry into the origins of the coronavirus and the world response, relations with China have been strained. At the core of the tension is an ideological impasse between liberal democratic countries and the communist government of China. To proponents of liberal democracies, China's strict censorship is ideologically deplorable and because this led to the cover up of the severity of the virus early in its emergence, some countries such as the USA have tried to blame China for the global toll of the virus. These ideological differences are entrenched and difficult to surmount. However, cooperation is required if the world is to tackle such challenges as disease and environmental issues which cross international borders. Therefore, ideological differences will need to be laid aside, however staunch, in order to engage in pragmatic cooperation.

Cooperation is powerful yet not always easy to achieve. Political differences will ever present an obstacle to effective collaboration. Yet, as the problems we face in the world reveal ourselves more interconnected than before, we must rise to the challenge of pursuing ways of working together, realising that "nobody can get there unless everybody gets there."

Comment Set E

Comment 1

My personal opinion (not speaking for IBM) is that DRM [Digital Rights Management] is stupid, because it can never be effective, and it takes away existing rights of the consumer.

****

Comment 2

Digital files cannot be made uncopyable, any more than water can be made not wet.

****

Comment 3

Trusted systems presume that the consumer is dishonest.

****

Comment 4

Hoaxes use weaknesses in human behavior to ensure they are replicated and distributed. In other words, hoaxes prey on the Human Operating System.

****

Comment 5

It's baffling to me that the content industries don't look at the experience of the software industry in the 80's, when copy protection on software was widely tried, and just as widely rejected by consumers.

Task A: Essay Sample 7
Comment Set E

Computer systems are integral to modern life and our way of life is reliant on computer technology which expands our power to create, understand and work. However, this increased reliance on computer software leads us to increased vulnerability to those wishing to exploit our reliance. How do we find a balance between reliance on computer technology where our most personal information is stored and protection from those wishing to exploit this very fact?

The idea of data protection and the vulnerabilities we face when using software is particularly poignant when looking at the widespread use of social media. Recently, a hoax made headlines for creating hoax accounts that mimicked an individual's Facebook friend in an attempt to persuade the user to give away personal information which was then used to blackmail them for money. In particular, this hoax sent a message as a friend asking for help resetting a password, relying on our human nature to help a friend in need - highlighting that "hoaxes prey on the Human Operating System". This example also demonstrates the increasing advancement of hoaxes and their ability to tap into the human psyche to exploit it.

Privacy and security are therefore a key concern when using computer systems. However, it could be argued some privacy and security measures undermine our level of control and autonomy when using computer software. For example, a new Google Recaptcha tracks mouse movement to determine whether the activity is human. Many users are not aware this information is collected while browsing to further develop this software, and consent is not obtained to use this data in developing more robust software against computer bots. At a theoretical level, how dissimilar is the non-consensual use of data in this instance when compared to a hoax? Although the intentions are consumer protection, this arguably removes rights of the consumer in terms of control of data. At a basic level, this is not dissimilar to how hoaxes remove consumer control of data. Therefore, it is important that privacy and security measures involve the consumer, and transparency is always the primary concern.

Our vulnerabilities when using technology are evident and can be preyed upon by those wishing to exploit elements of human nature. It is evident the line between protection from those trying to use our data in a self-serving way and is grey. However, when designing systems to protect us from this, it is important the consumer is aware and in control of how their data is used.

Task A: Essay Sample 8
Comment Set E

Digital rights management is intended to maintain an equitable flow of revenue for companies and artists that produce software and material. The laws can sometimes serve to hinder companies as they miss the opportunity for free advertising. Further, strict licensing laws have encouraged streaming services, such as Spotify and Netflix, which act as disservice to their respective industries by controlling the content available.

People want to share media they have experienced. The lines between breaches in copyright laws and distribution between friends is relatively grey. For those who grew up in the age before Spotify, it was commonplace to burn CDs for personal use and to give to a friend. Often, these would be a compilation of songs that had been ripped from other CDs. This could be considered a form of free advertisement for artists, and is in stark contrast to burning 100 copies of a CD to undercut commercial enterprises selling the same CD. This can also be viewed from the point of software. Ableton, a digital audio workstation, allows people to record and produce music on their laptops. The program costs approximately 1000AUD. Many people illegally 'crack' the software so they can trial it. 'Cracked' versions do not allow users to upgrade the program and have various other shortcomings as compared to the legitimate program. It allows people to try the program though, and gives people an opportunity to see if it is worth the investment, albeit illegal. Without the ability to circumvent the licensing, there may be music that simply was not made, it may curb the future of a flourishing artist. It is understandable that the companies need to make a revenue for their product, but humans are opportunistic, and even if there are laws protecting the digital rights to software, it will be shared among people regardless.

The recent influx of streaming services dedicated to visual and audio media are operating to combat the digital licensing protection of artists. This creates two issues: firstly, the artists are not compensated appropriately for users to access their media, and two, it is diluting the breadth of options available to people who use these services. It is a common theme that people sit at home and spend more time scrolling through Netflix trying to find a show, rather than actually watching one. The quality of these shows, as evidenced by the time treading through trash, is quite poor. Licensing, in this sense, is simply restricting the content that people have available to them. Netflix is notoriously 'trashy' and lacks a lot of independent and thought-provoking cinema. Artists should be paid for their work, but mainstream works should not be funnelled into easily digested avenues for the public to consumer at large. Then we must consider the compensation of the artists. It should be obvious that this discussion is not considering mainstream artists, but more independent based artists. They are forced to tackle this new medium of advertising, and often their music is lost in the sheer number of other options. This is compounded by 'suggested' playlists, which never showcase independent artists. This leads to question how much they are actually able to profit from the monopolised services they are forced to advertise their music on. It is akin to a small sticker on a billboard, no one notices the sticker.

While some sort of digital rights protection is necessary, the distribution of material is inevitable; if it can be done, it will be done. This is especially true of industries, such as arts, where people are notoriously not financially stable.

Comment Set F

Comment 1

Diversity in the world is a basic characteristic of human society, and also the key condition for a lively and dynamic world as we see today.

****

Comment 2

Majority cultures have a tendency to create a homogeneous environment, possibly limiting the potential diverse opinions can provide.

Comment 3

Diversity poses various challenges in communication, from differences in language to differences in culture.

****

Comment 4

Diversity is not about how we differ. Diversity is about embracing one another's uniqueness.

Task A: Essay Sample 9
Comment Set F

Diversity is very prevalent in the world as we know it. From cultural, racial and religious diversities, these factors all contributes to the dynamic world in which we find ourselves in. While diversity can allow for uniqueness, issues in differences can arise. At the end of this all, diversity ultimately involves the bringing together of cultures which is beautiful.

Diversity allows for a sense of uniqueness among one another. Those of differing backgrounds, whether that be cultural, race or religious aspects, all provide a distinction among the human race. In almost every country of the world, different cultures are observed whereby different customs make up the traditions of the people. In Muslim populations for example, they dedicate the whole month to fast in order to feel closer to their God. This is their unique tradition and is followed by this group of people, but not common elsewhere. Others respect this tradition and allow for uniqueness and diversity to thrive.

While majority of the time, diversity brings a sense of uniqueness, issues in these differences can arise. Racism is very much still prevalent in this day and age. Following the 9/11 terrorist attack of 2001, discrimination and racism was seen towards individuals of Arabian, Muslim or middle eastern appearance. This was in act of fear and hatred. The problem is the ethnicity of each individual was seen to represent the entirety of their culture. Which is problematic in a culturally diverse population and can cause division, and be detrimental to the population. More support is needed and changes to be implemented to bring about equality for all.

Ultimately diversity allows the bringing together of cultures. All around the world this diversity is seen but very predominantly in developed countries such as Australia, whereby the traditions of these diverse cultures are embraced and welcomed. Chinese New Year is celebrated around the country, which brings cultures together to ultimately thrive in a diverse society.

In light of this recent discussion, it is imperative to highlight that while diversity allows for the proper functioning of society and bringing together of cultures, there are still issues that can arise regarding differences. Until these differences are completely broken down and equality is observed, then we will not function as a fully diverse society.

Comment Set G

Comment 1

A person can be intelligent without being educated and vice versa.

****

Comment 2

Intelligence plus character - that is the goal of true education.

****

Comment 3

Education does not increase your intelligence. It is the other way around.

****

Comment 4

Expensive education gives you a head start. Intelligence allows you to transcend a poor start in life.

****

Comment 5

Our care of the child should be governed not by the desire to make him learn things, but by the endeavour always to keep burning within him that light which is called intelligence.

Task A: Essay Sample 10
Comment Set G

"Intelligence plus character-that is the goal of true education"

The educational system, namely schools and universities, provides students with a means of acquiring knowledge and skills, which invite future opportunities in the work world and social mobility. However, true education has also endeavour to foster intelligence and character. Intelligence, attributes such as creativity, adaptability, independent learning, problem solving, are life-long skills which allow students to not only navigate the work world, but serve as productive members of society. In a similar vein, it is imperative for education to develop character by instilling positive values which promote social cohesion, provide character-building opportunities which allow the student to ascertain personal convictions and develop strong opinions, and encourage involvement in ameliorating the community. The infinitely malleable nature of the child, which has deep roots in education, must be capitalised by fostering intelligence and character.

Intelligence extends beyond the acquisition of knowledge towards the application of it. Contextualising difficult concepts pertains to a more holistic understanding and appreciation. It is encouraging to see education systems shying away from the traditional method of dictation and of "spoon-feeding" information to the students, of which induces passivity and stagnates learning, but rather adopt problem-based learning approaches. This includes practical classes for science, scenario-based learning, innovative computer simulations and even engaging classroom debates. To illustrate, many schools and universities incorporate a research experience, whereby students learn to innovatively apply their acquired knowledge to novel situations. Furthermore, education systems must accentuate the importance of "independent learning," a vital skill which transcends the academic sphere and applies to almost everything in life. By mustering the motivation and curiosity to consult textbooks, journal articles and webpages outside of classroom instruction, not only will the student develop the propensity to perpetuate new knowledge, but they will also develop a passion for learning. It is undeniable that developing intelligence sets the student up for lifelong learning; a goal of true education.

In addition, intelligence encompasses an element of creativity, guided by a greater awareness of society. The NSW Board of Studies recognised a deficiency in the syllabus in this respect, thereby rectifying it to incorporate more emphasis on critical thinking. For instance, in lieu of the rigid modules and strict guidelines, English has been revamped to highlight the "power of writing." Students must confront the moral paradigms of social issues such as censorship, intellectual property rights, inequality, injustice, recruiting higher order thinking to generate strong opinions on these issues. This exposes them to the 'real world' outside of their classrooms and textbooks, not only leading to greater social awareness but precipitating an element of personal growth. By taking a stance on such issues, students reinforce their own personal convictions, which prepares them to be well-informed members of society.

Finally, true education must be a guiding factor into character development. As school is the microcosm of society, the emphasis on positive values such as honesty, integrity and tolerance are paramount, as these values are likely to be retained throughout adulthood. True education extends beyond the academic sphere, and must provide a plethora of character-building opportunities. Extracurricular activities such as leadership in a prefect body, peer mentoring, volunteering for homeless initiatives, environment clean-ups days, teamwork in sports, all act in concert to crystallise a student's self-discovery. They discover who they are when they ascertaining their beliefs and convictions; whether they can tolerate injustice in society and how they can be contribute to ameliorate it. A prime example is 13 years old Gidion Goodon who, unable to tolerate the crippling parking fees of Sydney Children's Hospital, successfully petitioned for its reduction in 2016. This act, which showcases his admirable resolve, resulted in more hospital visits for patients. Thus, extracurricular opportunities not only enrich the educational experience, but allows growth and character development, leading to a conscientiously self-aware individual; the true goal of education.

To conclude, true education extends further than the acquisition of knowledge, it encompasses development of intelligence and character. The novel teaching approach adopted by many schools serve as an encouraging shift to advocate critical thinking, problem solving, independent learning and creativity, facilitating more holistic and in-depth understanding of concepts. Furthermore, intelligence is quantified by the ability to form strong opinions whereby the student will learn to make future well-informed decisions. Finally, true education must emphasise positive values which promote social cohesion, and grant extracurricular opportunities which not only allow them to explore their interests, but fosters personal growth and character development. Thus, building intelligence and character, the main objectives of true education, are essential to set up students are productive members of society.

Task A: Essay Sample 11
Comment Set G

Educated fool

Coinciding with the end of World War II and the economic boom in the late 20th century, the level of education has only been improving chronologically. The access of education has been more accessible than ever, evidently with the increase in sheer numbers of schools of all levels - primary, secondary schools and even Universities. With this said, it has been highly controversial whether the level of education directly impacts one's intelligence or their success in future career and life in general. While the antagonists may suggest that the high level of education results in intelligent person, and success in their career, it has been strongly suggested, backed by scientifical data, that the intelligence of a person is "pre-determined" from the irreversible effects of genetics.

The intelligence in terms of education can be determined as one's capability to interpret and absorb information effectively. As unfortunate as it may imply, a number of papers in reputational journals in the field of neuroscience has suggested that approximately 90% of performance of a students is determined by their intelligence. Among the experts in the field, they have agreed that it is undeniable that the genetics of the parents play a crucial role in determining the offspring's intelligence as illustrated in rodent experiments. This includes how fast a mouse can solve problems (efficiency), how long that specific information remains in their brain (memory), and the complexity of the problem (capability) that can be solved. These factors are determined by combination of number of genes that affect the development of brain. Unfortunately, this is why some students, no matter how much time they devote into studying, seems to be limited in what they can achieve.

However, many people still believe the level of education is a key factor in forming an intelligent individual, and is a centrifugal factor for one's general success in career and life. Although this statement may not be completely false, the meaning of intelligence if being misunderstood in here. As the quote suggests - “Expensive education gives you a head start. Intelligence allows you to transcend a poor start in life” - the high level of education does increase one's potential and aid in high educational performance, but that does not correlate to the increase in intelligence. Rather, the level of education could be translated into the opportunity an individual has, and it depends on the individual how they utilise this opportunity and translate this into their success.

It is undeniable that education is pivotal in terms of success of individual, the society, and the whole of mankind ultimately. It is, however, crucial to identify the difference between an intelligent man with a highly educated man. Every individual can be a highly-educated person, if they are fortunate enough to be in the appropriate environment and possess sufficient money to pay for the education. However, the intelligence is rather an innate factor that is coded into our DNA, passed from our parents and ancestors.

Task A: Essay Sample 12
Comment Set G

Judging someone's intelligence by their level of education and academic performance is something that we are taught from the time we first enter school. Some people would define intelligence as the ability to learn, acquire and use new knowledge and we often associate highly-educated people with intelligence. It seems natural to think that highly intelligent people would receive more educat on as they would thrive in an academic environment.

But many people would agree that intelligence goes beyond your academic status or how much education you have received. A person may develop skills naturally through experience and may not require education to increase their knowledge. For example, if we take a look at skills required by employers when recruiting for new employees there are some skills, such as good communication skills, that cannot be taught but learnt through experience with interacting others. This shows that experience and self-reflection is as important in increasing your intelligence and it does not rely on education alone.

We also associate intelligence with how smart people are. Some studies performed by psychologists have shown that cognitive ability is not increased by education. This means that intelligence is not something that can be developed through being an academic environment, although being intelligent would give you a head start than others, most intelligent people would have this ability from birth.

There is a lot of debate on how we define intelligence and as Martin Luther King Jr suggests in the quote, true education lies more than just spreading knowledge. It is not just the academic skills that are required in intelligence, but it also can include the ability to interact and communicate with others and being able to persevere through difficulty without being discouraged. These skills would be learnt outside the academic environment and would not depend on how much education a person receives, therefore in this sense, as Kanazawa suggests education does not increase your level of intelligence.

Comment Set H

Comment 1

Democracy is an abuse of statistics.

****

Comment 2

Government, even in its best state, is but a necessary evil; in its worst state, an intolerable one.

Thomas Paine

****

Comment 3

Freedom is when the people can speak, democracy is when the government listens.

****

Comment 4

The worst thing in this world, next to anarchy, is government.

****

Comment 5

As I would not be a slave, so I would not be a master. This expresses my idea of democracy.

Task A: Essay Sample 13
Comment Set H

In today's given world, there are many developed nations that are deemed successful based on their GDP index or their people's income growth. Big players around the world like China, India and America often stand out as they are able to conquer a huge portion of the world's market due to their sheer size and economic developments they bring about as a nation. However, it is not always because of the way these nations lead their people that results in them holding important positions in the world market. Not all players, including these big players, rule their people in a democratic manner. Some choose communism and some choose anarchy and others may claim that they are democratic when they are not truly one. Democracy is essential to lead a nation to greater progress as its people feel valued and listened to.

An example would be Australia. Australia is generally viewed as a democratic nation where political decisions are centered on the view points and welfare of its people. True enough, the government did listen to its people when it recently legalised same-sex marriages. Although the decision to marry a person of one's choice may seem like a basic freedom one ought to have, the Australian government played it very beautifully by giving out a hidden message that the government does listen to its people who voice out their concerns. Legalising same gender marriages at a time where many nations around still hold a strong conservative viewpoint about homosexuality did show that Australia is truly a democratic country and one which understands the needs and wants of its people. Many people were elated and when people realise that their voices are heard, they are more likely to trust the leadership in the government.

On the contrary, there are countries who claim to be democratic but outrightly fail to listen and understand its people. One classic example would be the all-great America. The recent Florida shooting which has left 17 people, mostly students, dead is a huge signal for the country to ban gun control. Many parents and teachers have gone to streets to hold protests against gun laws and ownership. Parents of dead children are voicing their opinions in pain and agony. Despite solving this problem which has been an issue for many years and taking away innocent lives for nothing, the President chooses not to listen to its people citing a basic Amendment of the Law as a reason and deciding that instead of banning people from owning guns, he chooses to give bonuses to teachers to hold guns. A leader of a democratic nation is responsible for uniting and not dividing its people, not making a decision where the voices of the people are blatantly disregarded. This is not democracy, not the democracy which a great nation like America should follow.

In conclusion, democracy is most valued when people feel like they have been listened to and the government plays an active role to formulate policies to suit its people. However, the government should not only base its judgements on populace views but views that are important to the country in a long run. When the need for such policies arises, the government should take the time to explain to its people why such decisions are made and the impact it will have in the long run. Singapore, despite raising its goods and services tax by 2% took two parliament sittings to explain why such a raise was important even though its leaders knew that its people were unhappy about it. As such, it is always important to strike a balance between hearing the people's voice and formulating non-populace decisions for the greater good of the nation. It is only then that true democracy has been achieved.

Task A: Essay Sample 14
Comment Set H

Would the world be a better place without government?

People have been debating government versus self-rule since the agricultural revolution. Many argue that government provides structure and security, while others contend that government only serves to control them. I believe that while anarchy offers opportunities and freedom of expression, this is outweighed by the side effects of violence and neglect that comes with it.

Democracy keeps us safe. This key argument in support of the democratic system over the anarchist one focuses on legislation. Laws prevent the majority of citizens committing violent or harmful acts against others. Enforced by police, it is a relatively effective system. If a perpetrator wanted money to buy a new car and decided to rob a convenience store, they would have to consider the risk of serving years in prison and consider whether this was worth it for some new transport. Many people are discouraged from such acts by the mere consideration of consequence. Further, if the store was in fact robbed then the owner could be comforted firstly by the knowledge that people are looking for the perpetrator, and secondly that they may be reimbursed by their insurer (if they have insurance). In this way, people may have to work harder for the earnings, but at least they are protected.

Anarchy keeps us free. This is the core of the anarchical argument, that it is the ultimate liberation. All decisions are in the hands of the individual, with no restrictions or retributions from an overbearing government. If an individual believes that clothing is contributing to the body shaming culture of the modern day, they are free to walk around naked. If a poor family wants to take their children to live on the local beach instead of in a stuffy counsel housing flat, eating the fish they catch and sleeping under the stars, they may do so. In this way, people who are born into a low socioeconomic status or those with counter culture views are able to take action without oppression from a government demanding that they remain quietly between the lines and use the ladder provided to make their way to a better life.

It takes one sour strawberry to ruin the punnet. This analogy relates to the idea that in an anarchist system, only one individual need has a desire to do harm upon others for the entire system to collapse. One person with their finger on the trigger of a gun can end the lives of thousands of peace seekers. When Adolf Hitler broke down the German government to instil anarchy, this is exactly what happened. These were such sanguineous times not because everybody was being avaricious or violent, but because only a select few were. The result was people begging for new leadership, and Hitler was ready with his Brown Coats to provide it.

Democracy keeps people safe from citizen abuse while anarchy keeps people safe from government abuse. Although the latter may offer greater opportunities for the lower class and allow people to express their alternative views more freely, it makes everyone vulnerable to the actions of the malicious few. I believe that the initial offer of opportunities and freedom of expression are outweighed by the risk of violence and abuse, which are effectively managed by democratic rule.

Comment Set I

Comment 1

Only when the last tree has died and the last river been poisoned and the last fish been caught will we realise we cannot eat money.

****

Comment 2

Environmentally friendly cars will soon cease to be an option. . . they will become a necessity.

****

Comment 3

I would feel more optimistic about a bright future for man if he spent less time proving that he can outwit Nature and more time tasting her sweetness and respecting her seniority.

****

Comment 4

Every human has a fundamental right to an environment of quality that permits a life of dignity and well-being.

****

Comment 5

After one look at this planet any visitor from outer space would say "I want to see the manager".

Task A: Essay Sample 15
Comment Set I

Environmentalists have long been advocating for and demanding change with regards to the way we as a society treat the environment. From the use of plastic bags in grocery stores to the vehicles we drive on a daily basis it is clear that we as a population have impacted and altered the environment we live in. Technologies that are perceived as 'clean' have been developed and offer a more ecologically friendly alternative from traditional technologies. One such technology is the electric automobile. Australian families average around two vehicles per household. It is for this reason that electric cars should be subsidised by the government to be made financially affordable for the average Australian family.

Fujio Cho once said that 'Environmentally friendly cars will soon cease to be an option... they will become a necessity'. This is quite an ironic statement from the Chairman of Toyota inc. A car manufacturer whose product has impacted the environment on a global scale. Toyota, a Japanese car manufacturer has been in the fore front of trying to develop new technologies to make electric cars compete mainstream. There are many issues currently with electric cars when compared to the traditional diesel or petrol engine cars. Such issues include battery life, charging stations and affordability. Along with Toyota, Tesla is an American company founded by the entrepreneur Elon Musk. Tesla is often regarded as a paragon of what electric cars could potentially become in the mainstream market.

In Australia, currently the average price of a new Tesla car is approximately $100,000. Such a price is well out of the price range of the average Australian family. As Tesla is a private company, it maintains the right to price their product as they see fit. Pricing a product at such a high price has repercussions. If the Australian government were to invest in and subsidise the purchase of electric cars, they would become more affordable for the average Australian. Such an investment is not cheap to say the least. In saying this however, if the majority of Australians started to purchase electric cars, then other vehicle manufacturers would have a greater incentive to invest and continue to develop in greener technologies for their products.

Opponents of such a proposal would quickly highlight the enormous cost of such a program. Further analysis would have to be conducted to understand the exact pricing required and the overall benefit such a program would have on cutting emissions.

It is clear that human beings and especially automobiles have had a large impact on the environment. It is for this reason that there should be a shift towards greener technologies. Electronic cars should not be seen as a luxury item but rather as a technology that is clean and has the potential to improve the effects human beings have has on the environment.

Task A: Essay Sample 16
Comment Set I

"Only when the last tree has died and the last river been poisoned and the last fish been caught do we realise we cannot eat money"- Indian Cree Proverb

The debate on climate change is one of the most polarising issues of the 21st century. While scientific evidence points towards global warming being an alarming reality attributed to human actions, climate change sceptics dismiss this, claiming such temperature fluctuations are part of a natural cycle. Whether or not these claims derive from a desire to protect financial interests, it is undeniable that inactivity will only exacerbate the situation and cause substantial environmental damage. It is imperative that the environment, our quintessential source of life, must be protected at all costs because "only when the last tree has died and the last river been poisoned and the last fish been caught do we realise we cannot eat money." (Indian Cree Proverb)

Humans must firstly acknowledge their accountability for the damage they have already inflicted on the environment. Turn on the television and there are harrowing scenes of arctic animals struggling for life as rising temperatures destroy their habitat, of the horrific BP oil spill which poisoned so much sea life, of turtles choking on plastic bags. Climate scientists have warned of rising sea levels and global temperatures, as evidenced by 2017 being the hottest year and yielding the greatest air pollution on record. Furthermore, the increased carbon dioxide emission since the Industrial Revolution has been empirically observed from Antarctic ice core samples, thereby confirming that the culprit of global warming being the accumulation of greenhouse gases from vehicle exhausts and industrial sources. As the most self-aware and intellectually advanced beings on this planet, humans have the responsibility to protect the environment and ensure a life of dignity and well-being to future generations.

However, the evidence pertaining to climate change is still met with unprecedented scepticism. For instance, last year saw the shocking event of the United States President Donald Trump withdrawing from the Paris Accord; a worldwide climate change mitigation strategy which endeavoured to reduce the greenhouse gas emissions and minimise increases in global temperature. Despite the US being the second greatest emitter of carbon dioxide, following China, Trump maintained that the pollution taxes and emission reductions associated with the agreement would jeopardise the coal industry and undermine the US economy. Major corporations with financial investments in the coal industry also echo such sentiments, evidenced by ExxonMobil providing significant funding to mislead the trustworthiness of climate change science. While prioritising the "revitalisation of the coal industry" may yield short-term economic benefits, the long-term consequences of these actions must be considered. Namely the deleterious effect of the colossal industrial carbon emissions upon the already deteriorating environment.

While the financial motivations of these sceptics have led to regression on the climate change issue, it is encouraging to see worldwide progress on environmental protection. In particular, the Emissions Trading Scheme (ETS), an international trading mechanism, has been implemented to reduce carbon emission. This government-run, market-based approach allocates a number of permits to discharge specific quantities of greenhouse gases, thereby mitigating global warming and stimulating technological and economic growth. Moreover, certain innovations such as Google's self-driving environmentally friendly car have been developed to operate on electricity instead of unsustainable fossil fuels. While these cars are expensive, it would take government recognition of climate change to propel certain policies and ultimately render these cars economically viable. Additionally, there is still much that can be done on a local level; just be reducing our carbon footprint by taking public transport, recycling and utilising more sustainable energy sources such as solar power, we can all contribute to collectively reducing carbon emission. As global citizens, we all have an obligation to protect the environment and to protect life present and future; it is time to fight for the acceptance of climate change and take action against it.

In conclusion, while scientific evidence pertains towards the detrimental impact of climate change, the widespread scepticism against it, derived from the desire to protect financial interests, has stagnated progress on mitigation strategies. However, it is essential to prioritise long-term protection of the environment over the short-term economic benefits from the coal industry. The key to life is in protecting the environment, to fight for the acknowledgement of climate change, and to take responsibilities to rectify the damage now.

Task A: Essay Sample 17
Comment Set I

Have Global Strategies to Combat Environmental Pollution Been Effective?

William S. Burroughs remark that "After one look at this planet any visitor from outer space would say "I want to see the manager"" suggests that globally the environment is in a terrible state and dying at the hands of human exploitation. Certainly, global average temperatures have risen exponentially. In 2016 and 2017, the world's surface air temperature was recorded as being greater than 1 degree Celsius above pre-industrial levels for the first time. This has led to the inexorable rise of sea levels, caused by melting ice caps and the thermal expansion of sea water. The rise of modern technology has seen a dramatic increase in the number of factories and with greater economic success the underlying health of the environment has suffered drastically. Now the extent of the problem has been recognised, how is it being managed? Recent global strategies have so far proven to be largely ineffective.

The two major international agreements to resolve global environmental pollution have unfortunately adopted a myopic mindset. Firstly, the Kyoto agreement, which was signed by the majority of large nations in 1997, was widely agreed to have been unsuccessful. Essentially, specific targets were set in order to reduce carbon-based emissions. There were two main reasons why it ultimately proved inadequate. The first: India, and most notably China, as developing countries, weren't mandated to reduce emissions. The rationale that they contributed a relatively small share of carbon dioxide when the protocol was first initiated. The second reason was that the US didn't sign the treaty. By the time developments were in place, in 2005, US and China created more greenhouse gases to erase all of the reductions made by the others. In fact, emissions increased by 40% between 1990 and 2009.

Secondly, the Paris agreement has developed measures that aren't sufficient to make a significant change either. The main aim was climate change mitigation, specifically to hold the global average temperature at no more than 1.5 degrees Celsius above pre-industrial levels. Despite there being no concessions for developing nations (as per the Kyoto agreement), emission targets were separately negotiated for each country and voluntarily enforced. This lack of any punitive deterrence is insufficient to produce lasting change. In addition, US president Donald Trump ceased Us participation in June 2017, stating that it would be more beneficial for American business and workers outside of the agreement. They are currently engaged in a 4-year exit process. Again, no real punishment administered.

In spite of these shortcomings, there have been some positive steps taken to save the environment. In particular, China have made enormous progress in the last 4 years, since the Chinese Premier, Li Keqiang, declared war against pollution. There has been a reduction of 32% in fine particulates in air, as a city average. This has been achieved by very specific objectives: prohibiting new coal-fired power plants in the most polluted areas, reducing the number of cars on the road in the large cities, such as Beijing and Shanghai, and removing coal boilers from homes. These measures are an indication that significant changes can be made with a structured and focused approach. However, on a global scale, not enough is being done to rectify the environmental problems that have been created.

It is clear that recent measures have been largely ineffective. It is also clear that there are schemes that are working, such as many of the methods currently employed in China, and so improvements can be made with planning and sacrifice. Perhaps the only way to ensure lasting change in the future is to create strict penalties that are protected by global laws and world court to ensure recompense.

Comment Set J

Comment 1

The public good is in nothing more essentially interested, than in the protection of every individual's private rights.

Sir William Blackstone

****

Comment 2

In Republics, the great danger is that the majority may not sufficiently respect the rights of the minority.

James Madison

****

Comment 3

Individual rights are not subject to a public vote; a majority has no right to vote away the rights of a minority; the political function of rights is precisely to protect minorities from oppression by majorities (and the smallest minority on earth is the individual).

Ayn Rand

****

Comment 4

The majority is always wrong; the minority is rarely right.

Henrik Ibsen

****

Comment 5

If the measures which have been pursued are approved by the majority, it is the duty of the minority to acquiesce and conform.

Thomas Jefferson

Task A: Essay Sample 18
Comment Set J

Rarely in political situations are unanimous decisions made. Minority opposition to particular points of contention are inevitable and it is the role of governments to navigate the rocky and treacherous seas of public opinion and to arrive at a destination appreciated by all. This is not easy to do and undoubtedly there will be large bodies of people who disagree. But as long as the rights and freedom of all people are considered in the decision-making process, decision which favours the majority of public opinion are the right ones to make.

It goes without saying, governments must respect the rights and freedoms of every individual. Protection of these rights are the sole responsibility of governments. As Lord Acton famously states: "Liberty is not a means to a higher political end. It is itself the highest political end". The constancy of human progress throughout history has been towards the end of freedom and irresponsible governments that corrupt and abuse the power bestowed to them are not only doomed to failure but also represent a return to savagery. Thus, while a majority rule may present a clear decision, the majority cannot stifle out the universally accepted individual rights. Often tyrannies of many are not much better than a tyranny of one.

However, the protection of rights has no relevance to the submission to public opinion. While rights are concrete, universally accepted and protected by law. Public opinion is a dangerous, unpredictable beast, prone to sudden and extreme mood swings and influenced not by concrete, supporting values and morals, but by social media, television, advertisements, acts of popularity and other endeavours that attempt to seize public attention.

For this reason, complete obedience to public opinion in policy making and decision processes is no way to run a government. Such a government would be unstable, leadership and party ideals would be in constant turmoil and the resulting decisions made would be contradictory to reflect this. Several democracies in the world today reflect this, Australia and the UK to name a few. Such governments stagnate and halt completely, something perhaps even worse than making a decision not completely supported by the public.

How then are governments expected to lead such an unruly, divided and often confused society? Whilst public opinion is not reflective of the true values of many citizens, a majority in public opinion is the only concrete way to make a decision. In these cases, governments must strive to appease as many members of the community as possible, consider the needs and desires of all stakeholders, prioritise in terms of urgency and importance and then choose a course of action that seems to align with most of public opinion. If careful and due consideration has been given, those of the minority must "acquiesce and conform" as Thomas Jefferson states, if a decision is to be made at all.

This is not to say that the decisions made by the majority are always the right decisions to be made. They often are not and all governments are liable to make many mistakes in their lifetime, eliciting countless occasions of reform. However, this democratic method of government is the most reliable in maintenance of the liberties of the individual. It is thus the duty of all people to constantly keep our governments in check, to remain politically active and to exercise our right to speech and opinion.

Decisions made by the majority are often the best path of action, better than no course of action or a course of action completely departed from public opinion. In such decisions aligned with the majority public opinion, it is our duty to accept the decision but continue to strive for improvement.

Task A: Essay Sample 19
Comment Set J

Is imposing the will of the majority fair?

One of the standards that modern countries evaluate themselves by is the state of their political systems. It is considered the modern and fair way to govern a society is by allowing them to ultimately control what happens to that society. The democratic process is one that should involve everyone having an equal say and the majority rules. Therein, however, lies the problem. Possibly then this means that people who are in a minority risk being unheard, perhaps oppressed and disenfranchised. Is it fair that anyone in a modern society should be made to go against the grain of their own opinion? I think so and I believe the current pandemic provides the best argument to demonstrate this.

As we are all painfully aware the world is in the grip of a pandemic. Covid-19 has spread worldwide and the global death toll has just passed 1 million. Here in the UK the government who have been voted in by a democratic process have been trying to control the spread of the virus by introducing restrictions on social gatherings, opening of businesses and generally how we interact with others. Since the original lockdown that began in March there has been increasing anger and mistrust brewing in a minority of the population. Words like conspiracy and 'plan-demic' have been popping up more frequently on social media and in main stream media as well. These range from those who believe the virus doesn't actually exist at all and has been a construct to control the population at large, to those that just don't want to be told they have to wear a face mask. My point here is that they are certainly entitled to their opinion, but in this particular case if they were allowed to carry on with their lives the way they wanted to, we all would suffer. Opinion is different to fact, and the medical data is undeniable, but there are many who disregard this data by calling it a smear campaign to scare us into inevitable control. How do you argue with that, you can't reason with the unreasonable. The issue here is the greater good.

I realise that there is a danger in a democracy for race or religious minority groups to be suppressed. That is something that I certainly do not condone, and it is important in any healthy democracy that there is open and transparent debate and processes to prevent this from happening. I fear, however, that people confuse democracy with their right to do whatever it is they feel they should be able to. If the majority didn't conform and follow guidelines like social distancing then it would be the vulnerable in society that will pay the price with this deadly virus. Perhaps with their lives.

Therefore, I have to agree with Thomas Jefferson who said 'if the measures which have been pursued are approved by the majority, it is the duty of the minority to acquiesce and conform.' In this particular time in our history the majority must rule, our lives may just depend on it!

Comment Set K

Comment 1

Whoever said the pen is mightier than the sword obviously never encountered automatic weapons.

Gen. Douglas MacArthur

****

Comment 2

Political power grows out of the barrel of a gun.

Chairman Mao Zedong

****

Comment 3

The most foolish mistake we could possibly make would be to allow the subject races to possess arms.

Adolf Hitler

****

Comment 4

Before a standing army can rule, the people must be disarmed, as they are in almost every country in Europe.

Noah Webster

****

Comment 5

You can get more with a kind word and a gun than you can with just a kind word.

Al Capone

Task A: Essay Sample 20
Comment Set K

Mankind's desire for power has been a feature throughout our whole human history. From the days of competing clan's millennia ago to today's modern inter-state and intra-state political power struggles. Such competition often drives technological advancements in weaponry that can be the key to victory. However, does this method actually ensure the best and most fair outcome? Is our use of force and weaponry outdated? Have we not seen enough unfruitful displays of war and death to realise that this should not be the way for human progress?

The level of human innovation and invention goes far beyond that of weaponry such as guns. Our species, has managed to do what very few other animals have ever been able to do. Through sophisticated language and communication, we have the ability to work together on a mass scale - with the ability to apply reason and thought in order to ensure better outcomes. Surely, this is a far better weapon than any advancement that gives us the ability to kill and harm one another. If not, are we not simply as primal as wild animals? "Whoever said the pen is mightier that the sword obviously never encountered automatic weapons" was a famous comment made by Gen. Douglas MacArthur. This precise mindless attitude displays complete disregard for the power of communication and importance for it. According to Steven Pinker book, 'The better angels of our nature' that contrary to what we see and read from mass media, we are in fact living in the most peaceful period in our human history. This phenomenon has not come about through mass suppression through force and weaponry, it has developed through better communication as a species, leading to greater democratisation and freedom.

An appreciation however, must be given to certain points in history where it could be argued that battle and war was the only option. The world at the start of the twentieth century led us to great rises in nationalistic mindsets with the thirst for power at all costs. During both world wars force was indeed necessary to defeat the tainted ideologies of a few. Whilst a case can be made that force is necessary on occasions, it should never be the first and definitely not the only option. As when this mentality become the norm, individuals can see that as the only way to gain power. No more evident than with Chairman Mao Zedong - "political power grows out of the barrel of a gun".

We must as a society adapt to the times we are living in. We live in a world where we are more connected than ever. Where we can learn and understand people and cultures from all over the planet. This must lead us to better communication rather than simply fighting. In a world today, where we are faced with some global humanitarian crises such as global warming, our attention must be focused here rather than looking to hurt and fight one another.

Comment Set L

Comment 1

Make the Revolution a parent of settlement, and not a nursery of future revolutions.

Edmund Burke

****

Comment 2

In some cases nonviolence requires more militancy than violence.

Cesar Chavez

****

Comment 3

The first duty of a revolutionary is to get away with it.

Abbie Hoffman

****

Comment 4

If we behave like those on the other side, then we are the other side. Instead of changing the world, all we'll achieve is a reflection of the one we want to destroy.

Jean Genet

****

Comment 5

When liberty comes with hands dabbled in blood it is hard to shake hands with her.

Oscar Wilde

Task A: Essay Sample 21
Comment Set L

"If we behave like those on the other side, then we are the other side. Instead of changing the world, all we'll achieve is a reflection of the one we want to destroy" - Jean Genet

Revolutions are a means of instigating radical social change or political reform, often by resistance against oppressive authorities. People who have suffered abuse, exploitation, oppression or discrimination often seek to rectify their situation by attempting to win freedom, equality and justice by force. Although such revolutions are a means of being heard, this violence ultimately corrupts the soul and perpetuates itself; the revolutionaries reflect the values which they have fought against. This is encapsulated in Jean Genet's quote "if we behave like those on the other side, then we are the other side. Instead of changing the world, all we'll achieve is a reflection of the one we want to destroy." Thus, while revolution demands a disturbance of order to enact change, violence is not necessary to achieve these aims.

Employing violence to take freedom by force only poisons the soul. Using negotiation and non-violent protests can catalyse revolution without compromising one's integrity and moral standards. Mahatma Gandhi, the leader of the pivotal independence movement in British ruled India advocated nonviolent civil disobedience, thereby instilling values of peace and resolution as he guided the nation towards independence. His methods included long fasts to protest and marches to protests against the subjugation of the disadvantaged classes, and the injustices that the British inflicted upon the Indian people, of whom were deprived of their rights. In the Salt March of 1930, he led hundreds of thousands of Indians on a 240 miles march to collect salt from the Arabian Sea, as a demonstration of disobedience against the British monopoly on salt trade. Despite the fact that 60,000 Indians were imprisoned on the journey, it was a demonstration of immutable courage and solidarity from people who willingly elevated the love and pride for their country above their own lives. Eventually, the British granted India their salt rights again. Furthermore, after Gandhi was imprisoned for his "Quit India" speech regarding India's independence from British rule, millions of people all over the nation held massive protests and non-violent demonstrations for his release, of which was testament to Gandhi's influence. The phenomenon caused Britain to relinquish its grasp on India in 1942, thereby proving that non-violent measures can achieve revolutions without regression of human morality.

However, many would argue that violence is necessary for the success of a revolution. The French Revolution of 1789-1799 was a far-reaching political upheaval which employed force and violence to overthrow the monarchy. The perceived order within the country was a guise for resigned compliance to oppression, in fear of persecution; violent revolution was a means for people's voices to be heard. The Revolution led to an abolishment of the feudal system, emancipation of the individual and establishment of equality. It was a unreckonable movement which was also instrumental in triggering a global decline of absolute monarchies, thereby ameliorating the quality of life for oppressed people everywhere. To further illustrate, the heavily censored non-violent Tiananmen Square protests of 1989 resulted in unforgivable, devastating massacres of the protestors that proved that the Communist party was complicit in crimes against humanity. Students who opposed the instability of a post-Mao era gathered in Tiananmen Square to protest for greater democracy, government accountability, less censorship and more freedom of speech. Such ideals were regarded as political disturbance, so the Communist governments enacted martial law and commissioned troops to apply force against the protestors. The relentless firing of ammunition from tanks against the unarmed, innocent civilians, was inexcusable murder in cold blood; more than 10,000 students, who had so much unfulfilled potential in their lives ahead of them, were killed. The lack of remorse from China's government triggered global outrage at the transgression of morality. Thus, violence is sometimes necessary to succeed in Revolution, as exemplified by this devastating chapter of history.

It is worth noting that should violence successfully achieve revolution, while it appears that revolutionaries are the victors, violence corrupts the soul and continually perpetuates itself. The arrogance derived from the immense power of destroying the opponents only beckons arrogance, of which is the driver of hatred and division. Once it gains momentum, violence never stops and will only perpetuate itself; the revolutionaries who will enact political reform will rule the nation by dictatorship, thereby eradicating the values of freedom, equality and justice that the revolution once stood for. Violence only achieves a reflection of what the revolutionaries wanted to destroy, and ultimately fails in execution.

Thus, although revolutions demand a disturbance of order to instigate change, it is possible to use non-violent measures to achieve aims, especially if protestors demonstrate immutable solidarity, courage and love for their nation. Violence, which although seems necessary to successfully overhaul governments and establish new orders, ultimately is a vice which poisons and corrupts the soul and continually perpetuates itself. In compromising one's integrity and moral standards, the values that the revolution initially stood for will have disintegrated, thereby reinforcing Jean Genet's quote that "instead of changing the world, all we'll achieve is a reflection of the one we want to destroy.

Task A: Essay Sample 22
Comment Set L

The origin of a revolution is for change, a good change. When corruption and injustice reign in a nation, the people must act. The objective must be for the people to be unshackled from the chains of inequality and strive for liberty, and ultimately, the pursuit of happiness.

Revolutions have occurred in many stages if history for the pure reason of disdain and unfairness of the people against the governance of the country. Revolutions aim in restoring equal law and order for all levels of citizens and to give opportunities for anyone in a society to live in liberty and happiness. There have been many revolutions against injustices in the social system, such as the Haiti revolution against slavery, and the French revolutions against corruption and poverty. The American Revolution marked the independence of the United States from the British rule, and help lay the foundations of a great nation that enjoys freedom and wealth for the last 200 years. The reasons for many revolutions were demands of freedom from oppression and to govern and prosper for the nation rather than being taken away by a coloniser or an oppressive government.

It is imperative for revolutions to be coordinated and led by pragmatic leaders who must control the movement as to ensure the image of the revolution is not hypocritical and not a mirror-image of their own oppressors. Egypt, in 2012, had its first "democratically-elected" government; the once "terrorist-branded" Muslim Brotherhood, led by Dr Mohamed Morsi. Besides the background of the brotherhood party, this was the opportunity to see if the "brotherhood" had the resources and values to lead the nation. Instead of sharing power with the parliament, Morsi began a tirade of "power grabbing", with some of his policies giving him absolute powers in regards to foreign policy, the economy and legal systems. H developed many opponents, such as one of the highest judges in Egypt. He soon came to resemble the previous Mubarak-era "totalitarian government". In June 2013, over 4 million Egyptian protested on the streets, and Morsi was toppled by the Egyptian military led by Field Marshal el Sisi.

If revolutions lose their focus and their initial objectives, then the foundations of the revolution will soon become fragile and will collapse until another revolution comes knocking in its place.

Leadership and keeping values are imperative for a revolution to stay legitimate in the eyes of the nation. Revolutions catalyse change in the political and social environment of a nation. We have seen many revolutions that have been coordinated and executed precisely, and this is due to the elements if liberty and justice acting as the banner for the movement. Revolutions can bring forth prosperity for a nation and lay down the foundation for future generations to enjoy. And let's hope that the revolution only becomes a legacy, not a living reality.

Comment Set M

Comment 1

If the past cannot teach the present and the father cannot teach the son, then history need not have bothered to go on, and the world has wasted a great deal of time.

Russell Hoban

****

Comment 2

The best of my education has come from the public library. . . my tuition fee is a bus fare and once in a while, five cents a day for an overdue book. You don't need to know very much to start with, if you know the way to the public library.

Lesley Conger

****

Comment 3

He who opens a school door, closes a prison.

Victor Hugo

****

Comment 4

Education is an ornament in prosperity and a refuge in adversity.

Aristotle

****

Comment 5

Education. . . has produced a vast population able to read but unable to distinguish what is worth reading.

G. M. Trevelyan

Task A: Essay Sample 23
Comment Set M

Does education significantly promote critical thinking?

John Dewey, the American philosopher and educational reformer, suggested that the purpose of education was to allow an individual to develop strategies and habits to discriminate tested beliefs from mere guesses. His theories still underpin much of the education that exists today. The idea of critical thinking makes sense: most of the revolutionary theories in science and the progress of civilisation are borne of critical thinking. It stimulated the ground-breaking ideas of Newton and Einstein, the evaluations of Darwin and the inspiration of Martin Luther King, Jr. These people did not accept what they were told or what others said was the truth. Each of them fundamentally shifted our worldview. But are current educational methods promoting critical thinking? A longitudinal study on divergent thinking (a central component of thinking critically) demonstrated that when tested as kindergartens, 98% of the study's subjects scored at the genius level. This fell precipitously to 32% at age 10 and to 10% by age 15 (Land et al, 98). Therefore, education does not significantly promote critical thinking and if anything reverses it.

Problem-solving at school is centred on trying to work out solutions to problems that have been neatly posed for students. This does not teach the crucial skill of identifying issues which in real life would not come packaged in this way. In the everyday world, the first and most difficult step in solving a problem is realising that one exists. When American car makers lost sales in competition with small Japanese vehicles in the 1980s, it was not that Americans had failed to solve the problem but they had failed to recognise it until it became apparent as a result of declining profits.

G.M. Trevelyan once said: "Education...has produced a vast population able to read but unable to distinguish what is worth reading". This is a true statement. Similarly, students are encouraged to solve all the problems that they are presented with. Critical thinking should revolve around teaching students that not all problems are worth solving. In real world situations the trick is choosing which ought to be solved and learning to ignore others. Trying to cope with all issues that arise can overwhelm us – students, scientists and business executives alike. For example, in 2015, large budget cuts for the Metropolitan police in the UK meant that radical reform of public safety was needed. Essentially, priorities had to be established: efforts into missing person cases and investigations into historical crime were reduced and focus on domestic abuse and shoplifting was increased. Distinguishing which problems are most important to solve is key to success in the majority of real-world issues.

There are some strategies currently employed in our educational system which do promote critical thinking. Everyday problem-solving often takes place as a group endeavour in which people behave differently and less rationally than they do as individuals. An example of where this group approach to critical thinking is being used effectively can be seen in the 'Problem-Based Learning' methods which form an integral component of many medical school programs. They help to develop lifelong learning skills and interdisciplinarity. In addition, students are encouraged to objectively analyse and evaluate an issue in order to form a judgement. Despite the success of these programs, the overwhelming weight of education, particularly in the crucial 5-18-years old bracket, is conspicuously devoid of promoting critical thinking.

So, we can see that the majority of strategies designed to stimulate critical thinking in education aren't effective. Some 'Problem-Based Learning' techniques do promote critical thinking but the majority of teaching particularly at school age is not successful in this regard. Moreover, we see that thinking critically can be the difference between success and failure in real world problems. Critical thinkers are able to make better strategic and more effective decisions based on the evidence they are presented with, not what they are told by others or assumptions they have made. Thinking in this way sets us apart from our peers and is an invaluable skill in everyday life.

Comment Set N

Comment 1

It is important that students bring a certain ragamuffin, barefoot irreverence to their studies; they are not here to worship what is known, but to question it.

Jacob Bronowski

****

Comment 2

Children have to be educated, but they have also to be left to educate themselves.

Abbé Dimnet

****

Comment 3

Often, when I am reading a good book, I stop and thank my teacher.

****

Comment 4

Intellectual freedom is the right of every individual to both seek and receive information from all points of view without restriction.

American Library Association

****

Comment 5

The dream begins with a teacher who believes in you, who tugs and pushes and leads you to the next plateau, sometimes poking you with a sharp stick called "truth."

Dan Rather

Task A: Essay Sample 24
Comment Set N

Education is crucial to human development; without learning, a human would not develop into what we would fully consider to be a human being. Unlike certain animals, whose behaviours are built in as 'instincts', much of what makes a human being must be learnt. As Abbe Dimnet said, 'Children have to be educated...' Henry Ward Beecher once said that 'ignorance is the womb of monsters.' It is true for example if we cannot learn to understand how others think and feel it is a source of much prejudice and avarice between people and nations. However, Abbe also added the caveat to her quote upon educating children, '...but they have also to be left to educate themselves.' There is much we must be taught, and much we must learn, but we must never be entirely willing, mindless receptacles for information.

The American Library Association says, 'Intellectual freedom is the right of every individual to both seek and receive information from all points of view without restriction.' This sentiment echoes Abbe Dimnet's sentiment, in stating the importance for varied input in learning, though it applies not just to children but to everyone. If education and learning is too linear, coming from a single source, or too prescriptive without room or opportunity to question, it is more than a shame, but a danger. Questioning the status quo is an essential element in positive change for a person and a society. Take the recent move in Saudi Arabia toward allowing women to drive. For a long time, women have been unable to drive automobiles in the country, and it is only through questioning what has been 'taught' that positive change and more equal opportunities for both genders can be worked towards.

The other side of the argument is evinced neatly when Isaac Newton said, 'I stand on the shoulders of giants.' He meant that all he had achieved, and it was a great deal, including much of the foundations of modern physics and calculus, was only possible because of everything others had learned before him. If one were to question everything, and seek out endless viewpoints and disagreements, it could become an impediment to progress and accomplishment rather than its aide. It could be argued that a child questioning the science he or she is taught could be beneficial to the extent it invigorates them to find the true source of the information, which might deepen their comprehension of the subject. But to question it beyond this point may damage their progress, if they refuse to accept what to a certain degree must be prescriptive learning.

Nevertheless, as Jacob Bronowski said, 'Students ... are not here to worship what is known, but to question it.' Without the freedom to seek other sources of information, and to learn to doubt and question, or those that have done so historically, we would not be where we are today. Take Charles Darwin, and his discovery of evolution. His discovery of evolution by natural selection went against the prescribed beliefs in a deeply Christian society that God made life, in lieu of a description which stated that life evolved through natural forces rather than divine intention. It is this ability to question that has underpinned many scientific, and political and social revolutions in human history, such as the movement toward racial and gender equalities we have seen over the last century or more in the UK and many other parts of the world.

In conclusion it is true that we must succumb to a certain degree of prescriptive education, and take in what we are taught, otherwise we would not learn or make progress. We must, as Isaac Newton did, have giants whose shoulders we can stand upon. Nevertheless, as it has been argued, the ability to question what is known, and to be responsible for our own learning and investigations, is every bit as important for a healthy society.

Task A: Essay Sample 25
Comment Set N

To what extent does education require an equal split between directly being taught content, and further individual self-exploration of this content away from a classroom setting?

There are many forms and styles of educating, ranging from basic rote learning and memorisation of concepts to problem-based learning whereby a scenario is presented and ideas must be pooled to solve it, honing and developing knowledge and skills in doing so. Schools and colleges are often torn between teaching content to students to improve their broader knowledge and understanding and teaching them specific facts tailored for better performance in assessment. This essay will aim to explore the differing views on how education should be balanced, and will provide a strong proposition for the need for individual effort outside of regimented classroom time.

'Children have to be educated, but they have also to be left to educate themselves' - Abbe Dimnet. Education and learning is something that cannot solely be delivered by a teacher. It involves, and requires, the equal effort of the student to want to learn, understand and develop the intellect. Subjects often taught in schooling systems are so broad and so extensive that they cannot nearly be adequately covered in a classroom in the limited time allocated to them. For a student to properly gain useful insight and appreciation for the field, they must invest time themselves to explore the themes and knowledge further. Teachers provide the basis and the platform for the students to then go away and elevate their knowledge to another level, and practice and enhance their skills, independent from their guidance. Some may argue that by allowing students to independently explore the avenues of learning, they are being left alone to unknowingly make mistakes, develop incorrect understanding and stray away from what is useful and beneficial for their education. They require constant guidance to ensure they develop, in an environment where mistakes are made clear and the right topics are provided for them. However, I would argue that making mistakes is one of the main forms of learning. Mistakes offer a unique opportunity to analyse incorrect methodology, appreciate the pitfalls and then improve. It is an often used saying that we learn more from our mistakes than we do our successes, as there is more to evaluate and understand in a mistake. Therefore I would suggest that making errors due to individual learning is not something to be feared, but rather embraced and welcomed, and it is a natural part of a good and worthwhile education.

Furthermore, schools and colleges have set criteria and syllabuses that they must follow when delivering lessons, seminars and lectures. They rarely allow room to stray into sub-topics and other areas that may interest certain students. Therefore, I propose that by allowing students to go away and learn more for themselves, we are promoting their broader education and exploration to other topics that they find interesting. Without the freedom and encouragement to delve deeper into different subjects, every student would be churned out the education system with the exact same textbook knowledge of everyone around them. It creates diversity, individuality and passions that mean we can benefit from the unique skills, know-how and interests of others in society. One could view unfavourably upon this and argue that by allowing students to stray away from the interests of the education system, they are distracted and not as focused on achieving the relevant knowledge and therefore qualifications required to achieve in life. The topics taught in schools have been chosen such as they provide the foundational intellect required for people to achieve in life. I would agree, but I think to suppress and confine students to the strict limits of a subject syllabus may actually do the same, promoting disinterest and leading to worse academic performance. Knowledge is power, and we must not prevent people from striving to gain more knowledge when they are interested to do so.

I strongly believe that there is only so much that a student can be taught and benefit from in a classroom. I think much of education involves the individual efforts of the student in identifying areas of improvement, and targeting them themselves. Teachers provide the crucial basis and foundations required to do this, and without self-education students will simply be confined to the mediocre basics of knowledge.

Comment Set O

Comment 1

People demand freedom of speech as a compensation for the freedom of thought which they seldom use.

Soren Kierkegaard

****

Comment 2

Freedom of speech means freedom for those who you despise, and freedom to express the most despicable views.

Alan Dershowitz

****

Comment 3

Social media is one big bathroom wall with people from all walks of life saying all kinds of stupidity.

****

Comment 4

True liberty means the right to tell people what they do not want to hear.

Task A: Essay Sample 26
Comment Set O

Does Freedom of Speech give humans the right to speak their mind absolutely?

The concept of freedom of speech is not a new one, in fact, it is quite an old one dating back to the ancient Greeks. However, I do understand the constant need to revisit its pros and re-evaluate its acceptable bounds in society. The unprecedented advancements in technology and social media continually pose a question on the morals of freedom of speech. We must not forget, however, that freedom of speech should not be interchangeable with freedom of thought and contrary to that as Soren Kierkegaard suggests, if we choose not to use our right to freedom of thought we must not expect to get away with voicing our opinions/beliefs if it means tampering with others' rights. Yes, you should be able to choose how to express yourself, but, in a way that does not incur legal consequences or interrupt the rights of other individuals. There is a myriad of reasons why the public fought for freedom of speech and the advantages that it creates acts as a testimony to this. Allowing society to speak up for themselves allows us to better our society in a peaceful manner. I can only speak for myself, but, I'd much rather the public use their voices rather than weapons. How many will disagree with this? Not many, I hope! I believe, freedom of speech allows individuals to, not only, express themselves but also learn how to be more accepting of how others choose to express themselves. We take for granted the ability to share with others, everything that we wish to.

Some will propose that any speech which offends others should be banned. The challenge is that everyone will have different thoughts on what offends them. Speaking out about gay marriage or gender dysphoria may offend people but, certainly, isn't a license to be banned. In particular, elderly people find It difficult talking about such topics as back in their youth it was frowned upon, but as the world and it's affairs evolves, we must let our minds evolve with it. As of May 2018, Blasphemy is no longer a constitutional offence. Saying something about god that others may deem disrespectful is now okay. I can see the pros and cons of this but, in the modern world we live in today, I think it's necessary for exceptions to be made for such arbitrary topics, otherwise we'd be here forever deciding what is and is not okay to say regarding religion and sacred things. John Lennon claiming that the Beatles were more popular than Jesus was deemed to be Blasphemy but I fail to see the harm in it. Of course there will be times when we wish others didn't have the right to say certain things but we must learn to not dwell in such situation but rather use them to teach ourselves to be more resilient.

Recent growths in social medica has opened a huge can of worms with regards to freedom of speech. The ability to reach thousands of other with the touch of a button is amazing until it's not. Unfortunately, there is very little safeguarding present for the things individuals are allowed to release on media. Bullying being a huge consequence. Bullying has been going on forever, however, now, cyber-bullying takes the problem to a new level. It is easier to say things behind a screen than to another's face. This is contradicting the bounds to free speech and, although, social media is great and wonderful, it can also be our demise. It provides an easy platform to making mistakes. If we say things online that we later regret, there is no means of retraction. Fake accounts and the very topical 'catfishing' is allowing people to violate the whole concept of free speech without being held accountable. I can just but hope as a society we aren't risking the need to have our rights seized from us due to such 'stupidity'.

There is some limit on the freedom of speech. Limiting free speech to public order and morality is absolutely necessary for our protection. Rightfully, we cannot use free speech to defame others as this would interfere with their rights. Like everything in life, if we wish to be respected, we must show respect. Same goes for rights. This is to say when used properly, freedom of speech can be a huge flex, as they say nowadays, of our society. Here, we meet our problem, we depend on the people using this right properly. We cannot guarantee that everyone will. Actually, we can easier guarantee someone won't. This is the sad truth about a lot of things in life. It is a matter of balancing the pros for those who will respect their rights and the consequences that will come from those who choose to contravene. If only it was as easy as allowing individuals to use their common sense, unfortunately, some people are lacking the sense they were born with.

The thing is, in order to protect our rights, we must respect them. The answer to my initial question, which I hope obvious at this stage, is no. We must not mistake our right to free speech as the right to voice every single thought and belief we have. If we do find ourselves having viewpoints that may offend or defame others, we must teach ourselves to be happy to keep these to ourselves.

Task A: Essay Sample 27
Comment Set O

The rapid growth of social media over the past century and its now found prominence in the Western political landscape has caused the debate over freedom of speech to heat up. The overpowering censorship of information and media posted on social platforms such as Twitter and Facebook have caused outcries from the public with claims that individual liberties are being deprived. Yet, censorship acts as a barrier of protection reducing the radical hate speech and minimising conflicts that could arise due to cultural and racial intolerances that paint the world today. While an ideal, absolute freedom of speech is not maintainable in society and accompanied by the speed at which media and information can travel from one end of the globe to another would result in chaos and conflicts. Instead, a balance must be found in which radical content is minimised and a tolerant society is fostered whilst still allowing enough freedom to raise societal issues and make changes to the current social structures which are oppressing the minority.

A world in which posts on social media are unmonitored would result in a world of chaos, intolerance, and conflict. Such effects have already been seen through Donald Trump's Twitter posts and their contribution to the Capitol Riots. His influential messages to the public lead to a violent and even deadly raid of the capital which with proper monitoring protocol may have been avoided. Left unchecked people are able to write hate speech, negative comments, bully and offend which on a smaller level can contribute to mental health issues and on a larger scale result in wars between religions, races or even countries. Worst of all this can be done anonymously in such a way that individuals can avoid any form of retribution for their actions. Such a world is unsustainable, and policies must be introduced to minimise these effects. Steps are already being made in this direction with Australia introducing new legislation to minimise the defamatory content by allowing victims to obtain the details of anonymous trollers. Such policies directly conflict with the ideas of freedom of speech and yet are necessary for the safety and sustainability of the current technologically advancing society.

However, it can still be argued that such censorship can actually contribute to the oppression of minority groups. Limiting the content regarding violence, for example the police brutality towards George Floyd would have completely extinguished the Black Lives Matter movement before it started. The actual release of such footage, which could be deemed inappropriate for media, was able to educate the world on an issue that was otherwise swept under the rug. It was this freedom of speech on social media that made the Black Lives Matter movement reach all ends of the globe with protests across not only the US but Australia and other neighbouring countries. Uncensored speech and media provide an avenue for oppressed to educate the majority on what is happening and fight for change. Limiting such power could contribute to a more stagnant society in which the repressed remain oppressed and the majority live in blissful ignorance.

As such, while absolute freedom of speech is not viable a balance must bs struck in which the minority are still able to express their opinions, challenges, and fight for change against the dominant social narratives that control society. The speed at which we can communicate globally has made this task 10 times more difficult and specific legislation must be implemented, in collaboration with the people, to establish the most appropriate solution.

Task A: Essay Sample 28
Comment Set O

Is what is our birthright always what is right?

Humans are proud creatures, and it is our innate nature to defend our values and beliefs that we hold close to our hearts. As a matter of fact, it is our innate ability to defend and safe-guard anything we hold close to us, period, whether it be our values or not. Imagine it sort of like a lioness protecting and safe-guarding her baby cub-that is the ferocity in which humans safe-guard their values, because there comes a point in time where out values become intermingled with our personalities and who we are as people. When situations such as this happens, it becomes a difficult path to take when it becomes our duty to speak against values that are morally and ethically wrong, or values which may be of danger to the society in which we are attempting to create. We may see freedom of speech as a choice of weapon to use, but it is in reality our birthright. The power of speech to challenge controversial beliefs is, as human beings, our rights. However, what happens when such defences and values go too far, in which we may seem to be causing more harm and healing by using our voice to speak up? As a result, the freedom of speech is a powerful weapon that gives humans the ability to speak up and challenge beliefs they believe to be detrimental to a society, but the power of speech itself can backfire and cause destruction and harm if not used with safety and thought.

Humans are a resilient species who has, in history, used their freedom of speech to challenge laws and rules highly accepted by the society in which they live in, to bring about social change. Without the power of speech and the liberty to speak our minds, history has seen much damage caused where people who believes their values are superior, have festered in societies like a disease, causing only harm on its pathway. Cries of the people are oppressed and ignored, due to their stubbornness and unwillingness to listen to the disadvantaged to safeguard their own values. However, if we do not continue to question such values and beliefs held by the cultures and religion and societies we have grown up in, how will we ever bring about change to the people around us? Peter Ellerton, Professor of pedagogy and physics at the University of Queensland, once said in his speech how a diversity of ideas marks a resilient society, and the capability to question other's ideas under critic and take in those critics without feeling attacked or offended is a sign of not only a truly resilient society, but also of one that is mature and growing. Take for instance the movement of the Suffragettes. If women have not marched or protested for the rights of women to vote, where will society be? Ruled by only the ideas of men in a political constitution, while women remain deprived of ideas and opportunities? Freedom of speech brings about equality, and that is by questioning what is difficult to question. As many have said in the past, "True liberty means the right to tell people what they do not want to hear." Professor Ellerton once even said that we cannot empathize with ideas as we empathize with people, as it is ideas that needs to be put under the microscope and examined for faults. Furthermore, if it was not for true liberty to speak out and protest against the mistreatment of black lives around the world, especially by the hands of police, then certain constitutional policies will never have surfaced. It takes a great deal of courage to question a department as prestigious as the police department, and most accusations of corruption were often dismissed due to the law-holders' prestigious political position. However, if it were not for the power of the people marching t demand justice for George Floyd and Breonna Taylor during the Black Lives Matter Movement, then the Breonna Taylor No Knock Policy, which is a huge step forward in protecting vulnerable lives from the powers of police enforcements, would certainly not have passed, and media coverage and support from around the world was what certain got the three police officers involved in Floyd's murder acquitted and charged. As a result, the liberty of speech pertains to question what is difficult to bring about change.

However, there comes certain situations when people may use the liberty of speech as a means of hate and as a means to spread misinformation. Misuse of many powers of the world has led to corruption, and the freedom of speech is most certainly one of them. History and even modern day are speckled with incidences in which friends, families, neighbours and relatives close to someone have used this powerful weapon to bring about harm to those around them. Propaganda is one of the main abuses of speech that comes to mind, and this has brought about much hate and corruption around the world. Hateful propaganda was certainly one of the reasons that fuelled the Christchurch shooting in New Zealand that killed many parishioners and church-goers, harming many innocent lives. One is forced to think of the hateful propaganda circulating during the era of the NAZIS regime, proving that even history bears the horrible scars of the abuse of the liberty of speech. As aforementioned, it is truly a dangerous weapon. Even in our modern day and age, people utilize such technology and social media to assert their questionable and misleading opinions in a way that can prove harmful to a society. Sure, social media is an ideal outlet for expressing thoughts and opinions and spreading valuable information. However, what happens when that information may seem to come from unreliable sources, causing chaos and panic in the wider community? An example is that of previous President Donald Trump during the time period of the 2020 COVID-19 pandemic, where he was spreading misinformation online, where it got so severe to the point that the ex-president was banned from the platform. Needless to say people were already in a complete frenzy, and what the world really did not need is an entitled political leader spreading misinformation that can indefinitely harm the public. As Soren Kierkegaard has said, "people demand freedom of speech as a compensation for the freedom of thought which they seldom use." As a result, the liberty of speech comes at a price, hence must be used wisely.

The liberty of speech is certainly a powerful yet fragile concept. With it you are able to bring about monumental change by challenging the values and beliefs of our leaders to question the laws put into place, and to demand to give back to the people justice. Nevertheless, misuses of this freedom of expression can be detrimental when to comes to dealing with propaganda as well as spreading misinformation. We must be wise in the way in which we use these rights placed upon us, and only use the liberty of speech to bring about change for the good of the society we are building, while doing no harm.

Comment Set P

Comment 1

Technology Today: a Modern-day Miracle or a Curse?

Task A: Essay Sample 29
Comment Set P

If someone from the future went back in time with the latest iPhone, they would be revered as a god. It would go against everything that the people of that time would have understood up until that point and would be seen as a form of magic. However, to anyone born now, the iPhone is a completely normal thing that is not even questioned, let alone revered. This mentality is seen everywhere throughout life. Things that used to be considered impossible have now become so commonplace that people do not even question what used to be. This mentality, while expected, can become a somewhat dangerous one. By taking things for granted and forgetting what it was like before certain technologies existed, the opportunity for complacency is able to root itself.

One example of a new technology that could be seen as an impossible magic in the past is vaccines. Before vaccines existed, people constantly died from a myriad of diseases that are now completely preventable today. At the time, it would have been a miracle to prevent these diseases and people would most likely do just about anything to get one of these 'miracle cures'. However, these times no longer exist in many developed countries and vaccines for a lot of those diseases now exist and are available. While this is incredible and showcases just how far technology and medicine has come, with it complacency also exists. This can be seen with the Covid-19 vaccination and the controversies surrounding it during the recent pandemic. The refusal to take the Covid-19 vaccine from such a large population of people worldwide showcases just how complacent some people have become with medicine and disease prevention as a whole. They forget what the world would be like without the magic of these vaccines because it is what they have known for such a long time. Even something as recent as polio and the worldwide collaboration to essentially eradicate polio via vaccinations has been forgotten or downplayed. This complacency that has been seen during the pandemic is just one example of how forgetting about how "today's technology is yesterday's magic" can become extremely dangerous and even deadly if not treated correctly.

That is not to say however that humanity should not evolve and continue to try and solve today's 'magic' in the fear of becoming complacent. There are still a myriad of problems across the world that do not seem to have any current possible solutions and could be described as needing a 'magical solution' to solve them. Does this mean that society should not focusing on fixing these solutions or developing the technology required to lessen their impacts in the fear that people will forget how we currently live? Of course not! Instead, the focus should be on finding ways to appreciate and cherish these solutions without losing sight of what was sacrificed in order to get there. Now this is often easier said than done as it is just human nature to adapt to new situations and look at the past with rose coloured glasses. However, while difficult it is not impossible and if more people started to remind themselves on how today's technology really is a form of magic, an appreciation for how far we have come could be achieved.

Comment Set Q

Comment 1

If nations don't think about the future, they won't have one.

****

Comment 2

As long as we do not learn from history, history will repeat itself.

****

Comment 3

To predict the future is to create it.

****

Comment 4

Future generations will remember past innovators that contributed more than just the miracles of technology

Task A: Essay Sample 30
Comment Set Q

The significance of history for the future: individual and societal reflections

History can influence individual and communal reflections that will be paramount to apply in the present and future. At an individual level, history can teach lessons to generate unique reflections. As the perspectives of individuals often affect collective perspectives and incite action to modify the future, reflections on past history become pivotal to influence and potentially encourage action. However, the information gathered from history may not always be a beneficial instrument for reflection and its application in the future. Nevertheless, this may be the result of a misrepresentation of history since an accurate representation would be likely effective to encourage future beneficial action.

From an individual perspective, history has significant potential to teach lessons and generate unique reflections shaped by personal experience, which may be paramount to influence the future. This notion was instrumental to philosophers like Friedrich Nietzsche, who emphasises the importance of applying history as a source of reflection and consequent enhancement of the present and future in his essay "The Uses and Abuses of History". In this essay, Nietzsche suggests that the revision of history should be directed towards gathering lessons to improve the present and future. Similarly, the personal reflection of the significance of past events can be explored through the literary work of Ana Frank. Her diary invites readers to imagine her experience as a young woman persecuted in Nazi Germany of the 20th Century. The stories of Ana Frank are likely to resonate uniquely for each reader, and to be shaped by each reader's experience of life, which may propel a unique assimilation of reflections to the readers' present and future life. The diary of Ana Frank will likely catalyse personal reflections about the significance of the atrocities of the Holocaust, and to fuel reflections to gather and apply lessons to current and future aspects of readers' lives.

Since individual perspectives compose the collective view, the collective perspective of history becomes relevant in its examination. History unites the members of groups and is likely to function as an enabler for communal reflection. Reflections gathered from history can give an account of previous events with which to elaborate and support the modern-day democratic policymaking which underlies the liberties and restrictions of Western societies. Since democracy is principled on equality, these regulations often encourage a certain degree of equality in society and are often focused on the provision of these principles to historically disadvantaged subgroups. The inexistence of historical documentation would likely decrease collective understanding of the histories of people, and of how this has shaped their modern-day existence. Consideration and reflection about the history of Aboriginal Australians as a subgroup largely impacted by a significant health gap is demonstrative of these notions. Since collective reflections have potentially influenced the views of political representatives, these reflections often translate into action, such as the elaboration of policymaking. Policymaking is likely to consider the decades of disadvantaged health outcomes of Aboriginal Australians, transmuted into a 72-year-old life expectancy compared to the average 82- year-old lifespan of their Western counterpart. Reflections and acknowledgment on the history of subgroups such as Aboriginal Australians was instrumental to shape modern-day regulations intended to bridge the gap. This example is suggestive of the importance of history to shape collective reflection to utterly lead towards action.

However, the lessons of history may not always lead towards reflection and consequential betterment of the future. An example of this was 'Whig History', name given to a practice in which certain historians wrote history in a way that was overly influenced by their contemporary political beliefs. In this kind of approach, events that did not seem relevant to them received little attention, resulting in a misleading portrayal of the past and of no use to the enhancement of the future. Nevertheless, 'Whig History' was the result of a corrupt depiction of history. A transparent discussion of history would not represent history as such. By this logic, a proper depiction of history and its reflection would still be relevant for individual and collective reflection and potential enhancement.

History is a source of reflection for individuals and communities. Since personal reflections often influence societal views and have the potential to incite action to enhance the future, the collective reflections of groups have the potential to influence collective action, such as elaboration of policymaking. However, history may not always result beneficial for the future. Nevertheless, this may not be likely to result from an accurate reflection of history. An accurate portray and reflection of history will likely have the potential instrument to propel future enhancement.

Comment Set R

Comment 1

We do need magic to transform our world. We carry all of the power we need inside ourselves.

****

Comment 2

The day I became a politician was the day I found magic.

****

Comment 3

The danger of believing in magic is believing it is real.

****

Comment 4

Today's technology is yesterday's magic.

Task A: Essay Sample 31
Comment Set R

Magic or truth?

What makes a magician's act so entertaining and awe-enthralling? It is the sudden and instantaneous change of pulling a rabbit out of hat that captivates the audience, but change that happens this quick is fleeting; real 'magic' is change from long-standing norms. To begin, in a modern world that is driven by innovation and seekers for answers, magic truly comes from internal power to see a problem and form a tangible solution. Furthermore, changes in social laws do not magically happen overnight, but come from courageous and persevering citizens who use their power of individual liberty to challenge social expectations. Evidently, magic is related to the supernatural, but taking tangible action by harnessing individual power is the true means of transforming the world.

Firstly, it takes more than mere superstitious beliefs for innovators to use the power of self-belief to achieve transformation in the modern world. Using this stance, as humanity evolved from the pressures of institutionalised thinking, such as the control of the Church's doctrines on our source of knowledge, freedom in intellectual capacity and outcomes increased. As a result, rather than relying on the superstitious ways of magic to change our understanding of existence, science became the utility to comprehend life on and beyond Earth. In particular, the innovative foundations of Isaac Newton's and Albert Einstein's work in physics, such as the Universal Law of Gravitation and the Laws of Motion, contributed to the development of NASA's modern-day space exploration programs and the establishment of the International Space Station (ISS). These include the Project Apollo (which put the first humans on the moon) and applying technology used on the ISS to develop Eye Tracking Device Equipment for surgeons to use in laser surgery on Earth. These achievements came from breaking the mentality of supernatural magic being the portal to transform the world, as sending people into space and placing buildings in orbit requires more than an instantaneous trick. Years of scientific development contributed to these momentous outcomes. As such, if modern humanity continued to believe such achievements were only possible due to the supernatural, we would regress into archaic mindsets, such as that of the people during the Salem Witch trials. Believing the devil had cast evil spells on young women (who may have been eccentrics of their time) led to the persecution, torture and death of many innocent lives. Magic can be fun and well- 2 meaning, but it also has damages if believing in it still carried through today. Thus, supernatural magic is not behind the transformation of the world, it is the power of individual knowledge that pushes humanity towards a new age of innovation.

Furthermore, transformation of social expectations requires more than superstitious spells, it is individual liberty that propels humanity towards change. When freedom of speech and expression of thought guide people's actions, they have more control over their outcomes and views on society. In particular, the Stonewall Riots in New York were a demonstration of gay rights, were demonstrators broke laws, such as assaulting police and damaging public property, but their unconformity was for a greater cause. Their actions paved the liberation of the LGBTQ community into the 20 th century. Evidently, harnessing the power of individual liberty saw pivotal outcomes, like US laws permitting same-sex marriage in 2015 and other countries, such as Australia, following in 2017. Magic could not have been able to drive such changes to the law or social stigmas that surrounded gay couples and marriage 100 years ago. It is tangible defiance – action – that propels society towards a new age of acceptance. This means all individuals have the power to become the change they want to see; to transform the world around them, which can lead to more open-minded thinking and an inclusive society. Hence, individual freedom holds more power than mere magic to positively transform who we are and see tangible success in the world.

In summary, magic can provide temporary awe and entertainment, but tangible and transformative change to occur takes more than an instantaneous act. Firstly, superstition does not hold the power to transform the world, it is the innovators and seekers for knowledge who have the solutions to our modern problems. Furthermore, wearing a collective cloak of individual freedom gives power to propel humanity towards positively transforming social norms. Magic yields in the light of true individual power.

Comment Set S

Comment 1

Only when the last tree has died and the last river been poisoned and the last fish been caught will we realise we cannot eat money.

Indian Cree Proverb

****

Comment 2

Environmentally friendly cars will soon cease to be an option. . . they will become a necessity.

Fujio Cho

****

Comment 3

I would feel more optimistic about a bright future for man if he spent less time proving that he can outwit Nature and more time tasting her sweetness and respecting her seniority.

Elwyn Brooks White

****

Comment 4

Every human has a fundamental right to an environment of quality that permits a life of dignity and well-being.

****

Comment 5

After one look at this planet any visitor from outer space would say "I want to see the manager".

William S. Burroughs

Task A: Essay Sample 32
Comment Set S

Environment, in which we reside plays an important role in food cycle and thus in turn, it has major role in human survival. Today, natural resources are depleting at enormous rate, global warming is at peak, it is a high time for citizens of global world to take immediate steps to save mother nature. Human beings are very selfish. They, for their own benefits can do anything. Detrimental impacts on nature are due to activities of humankind. But people are not aware about its counter effects, which are very harmful for their own survival. Also, every individual has a basic right to be in an environment which promise a life of dignity and well-being.

Curve of natural resources such as trees and rivers on number of existing and time graph shows decreasing at an exponential rate. This is alarming. People are becoming selfish without caring about their future generation. People knowingly or unknowingly about its long-term adverse impacts are cutting down trees in order to create more space to accommodate growing population of their own kind and create spacious shopping malls and luxurious building. Moreover, human beings always aim at leading easy lives. Aircon and refrigerators are the examples of such invention. They have become a necessity in all households. But people are not aware about the harmful chemicals they release in the outer world are going to negatively impact their own kind. Furthermore, some animals are the important part of food cycle. These animals are vulnerable or at the verge of extinction because of the global warming. This has hampered the cycle of sustainability to a greater degree.

Environmentalists play a vital role here, by making people aware about the actions that they should take in order to live healthy life and actions to make planet sustainable. People should not only leave this duty on government but also it is an individual responsibility as a citizen of planet. Cars which run on battery should only be an option and people should be encouraged to use public transport and carpooling. Also, people should take off all the negative thoughts about ruling a mother nature and instead, should enjoys the fruits that mother nature is offering and be grateful to her.

In conclusion, depletion of natural resources is a warning sign by earth that individual has to take an immediate further action. Even though, man has a right to live a life of dignity and his own choice, it does not mean that he makes unsustainable choices that not only affect others but also to him on long run. Nature has always been superior and human beings are part of it like other creatures. So, by thinking about exploiting nature for one's own benefit is cruel, and it will come back to them.

Task A: Essay Sample 33
Comment Set S

QUOTE: "After one look at this planet any visitor from outer space would say "I want to see the manager"

Planet Earth: Our Only Home

I remember learning about the solar system and all the planets as a child and I was mesmerised by the beauty of Earth. It was striking in comparison to all the other planets - royal blue and white. I just hope that my grandchildren will be able to enjoy everything our beautiful planet has to offer; the grandeur of our oceans, the luscious rivers, our sky-high mountains and evergreen rainforests. Unfortunately, the future of our home is in jeopardy due to our constant greed with money and advancement. As William S Burroughs said, "After one look at this planet any visitor from outer space would say "I want to see the manager"". There are a spectrum of man-made processes and items which have contributed to this global phenomenon however plastic is a major culprit.

Plastics - a groundbreaking invention just before World War II. It had the world in awe because of it's strength, versatility and affordability. We use it in food packaging, food preservation, homeware, technology, transport, weapons and even for medical devices and research. The production of our basic needs depend on plastic in this era. The issue with plastics is that it is man-made and takes more than millions of years to decompose. It is not biodegradable and it is filling up our land-fills and oceans. Wild-life in the sea are dying every second because of our selfish acts. Sadly, humans can be quite short-sighted. We make decisions based on temporary pleasure and gain and this has been supported by Psychologists repeatedly. Plastics are destroying our planet and we need to take action now to preserve what is left of our planet.

One would argue that we cannot survive in a world without plastic but we have to remember that such a world did exist. Plastic is part of our everyday lives and I understand that it cannot be discarded in an instance. Even this computer that I am using right now to my phone, water bottle and the chair that I sit on are made out of plastic. Plastic has made many items more affordable to mass produce. The recycling industry alone has created many jobs and we continue to fuel our economy thanks to plastics. Despite this, many items are not recycled properly.

Greta Thunberg refuses to get on a plane because of the fuel consumption involved and its environmental impacts yet we refuse to use alternatives to plastic. Many small businesses in Australia are using paper straws and encouraging the use of keep cups. It is comforting to see these initiatives and the current generation being conscious of the environment however this is sadly still a minority of the global population. Our planet Earth is our only home and we should treat it with the respect that it deserves. Being aware of the environmental impacts of our actions will help us make wiser choices. We need to look after our planet, because it is the only home we have.

Comment Set T

Comment 1

Nationalism is just racism with a flag

Peter Joseph

****

Comment 2

Nationalism is an infantile disease, it is the measles of mankind

Albert Einstein

****

Comment 3

Race, religion, ethnic pride does nothing but teach you how to hate people that you've never met

Doug Stanhope

****

Comment 4

And so, my fellow Americans; ask not what your country can do for you- ask what you can do for your country

JFK

Task A: Essay Sample 34
Comment Set T

Nationalism can be quite an allusive concept. However, it must not be thought of as synonymous with being patriotic. So what exactly is it and what is its significance? Essentially, nationalism describes the thought that members of a shared area, or 'nation' should have complete power over the ruling of itself. This idea is quite a modern one and prior to the 18th century identity was determined by varying factors. Before the renaissance the language of civilisation was contained to Latin, Greek or Persian. However, towards the end of the 18th century there was a shift in this idea of civilisation and people began to believe that identity was determined specifically by one's nationality. It was this point in time when people began to cast aside the ancient and began to speak and educate, only in their mother-tongue. This idea of identity being determined by your nationality progressed even further into the 20th century where the first real consequences of nationalism was observed and it began to become synonymous with segregation, racism and ignorance.

Following the end of World War I, German nationalism began to grow rapidly. This played into the hands of the infamous tyrant, Adolf Hitler, who used his gift of speech, to manipulate and deceive people into joining his political party. The war had left the German population in a severe depression and it was this which Hitler used as leverage to rally the German people. He blamed the Jewish population in Germany for this economic decline and poverty. This instilled a hatred towards Jewish people within Germany as many of the Jews remained wealthy whilst other Germans did not. This anti-Semitism or racism within the Nazi party was shrouded by a Nationalist idea that if it were not for the Jews, Germany would not be experiencing such difficult economic times. People became blinded by the continuous bombardment of nationalist ideas and believed that in order to regain their economic health they must rid the country of the "foreign entity". This notion that one small group within a society can be its downfall, epitomises Peter Joseph's comment, that nationalism is just racism with a flag. Take the Nazi flag for example. Physically speaking it was the identity of the party, a flag with an emblem. However, ask anyone today to identify this flag and it will turn up uncomfortable feelings. This is because what the flag symbolised far outweighed its physical responsibility. The flag is a symbol of white supremacy, hatred and racism. This racism and hatred was always a deeply rooted manifesto of the party. But, much like as Joseph says, the flag was somewhat like a mask, hiding the systemic racism behind a nationalist idea.

I think comment two aptly describes nationalism as a 'disease'. Einstein compares the idea of nationalism with that of a contagious affliction. During the period after World War one, extreme nationalism spread throughout Europe. The rise of Hitler and German nationalism was likely inspired by the plague of nationalist views sweeping through Europe at this time. In Italy, Benito Mussolini rose to power under the premise of solving the economic crisis within Italy at the time. Mussolini captured the minds of the Italian people through his powerful stature and speeches. His use of rhetoric and metaphors fuelled distrust towards socialist groups. Anyone whom showed liberal tendencies were beaten or murdered. The working class believed Mussolini's claims that their poverty was the result of the socialist parties and thus they supported him, for it was for the good of Italy as a nation. As these leaders began to arise and successfully come into power it encouraged a wave of nationalism both in Europe and further afield. The flood gates were opened, as such and allowed for extreme nationalism to infect many nations.

The use of the term 'infantile' is also an interesting one as it connotes something which is childish or occurs amongst babies or small children. It gives a sense that nationalism can be viewed as being childlike or frivolous. I think that there is indeed some truth in this, because if one examines the examples I have set out above, the underlining idea is that of an individual disagreeing with something and thus propagating fallacies about that thing so as to get his/her own way. This generalisation is much like how a child will throw a tantrum in order to receive or get what they desire. Hitler and Mussolini alike, craved power and thus used the notion of nationalism as a means to manipulate people into following them and thus getting what they wanted.

Nationalism must not be confused with that of patriotism or love of country. It is instead a degenerative disease which can take hold of populations and result in the spread of hatred, ignorance and segregation. We must remember this now more than ever, as this plight once again threatens Europe. We must remember that the danger and blame is not with those whom have possess different skin colour, political or religious belief or sexuality. The danger is with the child throwing the tantrum in pursuit of what they want... power.

Comment Set U

Comment 1

When you subsidise poverty and failure, you get more of both.

****

Comment 2

Everyone in society is better off when the poor and disadvantaged are given the support and resources they need.

****

Comment 3

Corporations and the wealthy get welfare, too; it just goes by other names.

****

Comment 4

Welfare should be a safety net, not a hammock.

Task A: Essay Sample 35
Comment Set U

It may seem that providing welfare does not help. People may become dependent on these subsidies and thus may be disinclined to use their own initiative to get ahead in life. However, welfare can also help a lot of people. There are those who are really disadvantaged and those who need some supplementary income during transition points in their lives. In addition, welfare can have the effect of benefiting all of society by creating the conditions for people to become better workers and also by ensuring more social stability. As such, even though it may seem that providing welfare does not help, it can benefit both individuals and society.

It may seem that providing welfare to people does not help them. This idea is promoted in popular culture as well as in politics. In popular culture, in Australia, there is the cultural iconography of the 'dole bludger'. This is the idea of someone who becomes so used to living off social security payments that they become complacent, and it becomes a way of life. Thus, they become disengaged from studying or trying to find a conventional job. Such sentiments, regarding the unhelpfulness of welfare to the individual, are also echoed in politics. A recent example, in Australia, was when Senator Michaela Cash said "...the best form of welfare is a job." when declining to support an increase to Centrelink payments in line with GDP. Such sentiments generally arise from conservative and neo-Liberal ideology which encourages the view that power lies within the individual. As such, the provision of welfare by the government is as an artificial intrusion into the personal lives of people, which inhibits their individual initiative and ability to achieve their full potentials. As such, in this view, welfare does not really help people

However, providing welfare can help a lot of people. Beyond cultural iconography and politicisation, there are people who are genuinely struggling to survive day-to-day, as well as those who are at transition points in their lives and need a temporary leg up. Firstly, there is the phenomenon of the 'working poor'. That is, people who are working full-time, yet are struggling to pay the rent and to put food on the table. This is most prevalent in the US, but such a situation is increasingly similar in Australia. Indeed, there is an increasing divide between rich home-owners and poorer home-renters. In this regard, supplementary welfare payments are very helpful in helping to afford daily necessities and living a decent life. Secondly, there are people who are at a particular transition point in their lives where welfare payments can be very helpful. For example, there are those who are in between jobs or those who are trying to pursue further education. In this regards, welfare payments can be a vital supplementary income for them whilst they find a more suitable job or whilst they are learning more skills. Indeed, most people seek to make the most of their lives, not live out their lives as 'dole bludgers'. As such, welfare has the potential to help a lot of people.

Furthermore, welfare not only helps individuals, but also society. As mentioned before, there are people who need to utilise the welfare safety net whilst they are finding a new job so that they can better put their skill sets to use. There are also those who use welfare whilst they are studying and learning new skills. Thus, welfare can help individuals become better workers, which then benefits the country's workforce as a whole. In addition, contrary to neo-Liberal suppositions, frequently in many societies, power does not lie with the individual, but with socially powerful groups. An example is the housing market. In recent years, around the world, existing home owners and investors, with their existing capital, have bought more and more properties, thus crowding out the property market and causing exponential increases in house prices. As such, individuals from non-property owning backgrounds, though they may be hard-workers, have been finding it increasingly difficult to afford their own home. In this regard, the provision of welfare, or subsidies, can be a way to help more people in society own their own home. This also helps stem a situation where there is an increasing transfer of wealth from renters to landlords. A cautionary lesson is the French revolution. In that situation, the governing, land-owning class drained so much wealth from the ordinary people, without giving anything back, that the later rose up and overthrew them. As such, the provision of welfare could have been a way to return wealth to the people, as well as to maintain a more egalitarian and stable society. Thus, welfare can be good for society by providing the necessary support for workers to reskill and contribute better to the workforce of a country, and it can also be a way to maintain a more equal and fair society.

In conclusion, although it may seem that welfare does not help, it can help both individuals and society at large. Cultural and political images may promote the belief that welfare makes people complacent and discourages them from utilising their own initiative to study, find a job, or otherwise get ahead in life. However, welfare does benefit individuals. Such people who benefit include those who are trying to survive day-to-day, or those who are in the midst of transitioning to new jobs to better fit their skill sets, or those who are learning new skills. Furthermore, welfare also benefits broader society. By providing welfare support to those in job transition, or who are studying some more, society benefits by having a more adept workforce. More broadly, welfare can serve to redistribute wealth from the rich and powerful to the poor and powerless in order to maintain a more stable society. As such, although welfare may seem to be unbeneficial, it can benefit both individuals and society.

Task A: Essay Sample 36
Comment Set U

QUOTE: “The true sign of intelligence is not knowledge but imagination.”

Creativity: A necessity for progress

Humans have thrived on Earth because of our ability to innovate and adapt to our constantly changing environment. We have developed this skill to the point where we are able to control many aspects of our constantly evolving world. Some humans have contributed to our progress more than others and while we may see them as more intelligent beings; it is their ability to create and their imagination that sets them apart as opposed to mere knowledge. Knowledge of the past can guide the future however this alone will leave us in a world without growth. Creativity needs to be at the forefront for civilisation to continue thriving.

One of the characteristics Dr Yuval Noah Harari uses in his book ‘Sapiens’ to distinguish Homo Sapiens from other species is our ability to imagine. Our imagination made up for other areas we lacked in terms of size and speed. Homo Sapiens made it to the top of the food chain because we were able to manipulate our surroundings and create tools which were key to our survival. The discovery of controlling fire gave us light; a method to cook food which we previously could not digest, and also gave us the opportunity to fend off predators. The ability to create tools also allowed us to maximise the dexterity of our hands. These discoveries are not made from knowledge alone, but imagination.

Steve Jobs and Bill Gates are well-known globally for their innovations in the technology industry, are regarded as some of the most intelligent men; however, they are both college drop outs. This fact is concerning as it seems that educational institutions and our current education system in general does not recognise intelligence as innovation and creativity. Schools still place a huge emphasis on rote-learning and base assessments around this. In an era where most people have easy access to Google, there is no need for human encyclopaedias. The ability to retain information may have been desirable in the past, but the drive to propel our future with new innovations is what is currently needed. Those who contribute to the society with medical, technological, and other creations allow for a better quality of life, and it is their creativity that deems them intelligent as opposed to pure knowledge.

What the world needs is people who think outside of the box to help us tackle issues such as global warming and chronic health conditions. Each remarkable innovation in history has paved the way for our future. Our education system needs to recognise this to begin instilling these qualities in children from a young age, so that we create intelligent adults. These intelligent beings will have solutions to arising problems of the future. We need to allow our children to draw, create, play dress-up, dream, and imagine for a better future. Knowledge alone will not cut it.

Comment Set V

Comment 1

If you carry your childhood with you, you never become older

****

Comment 2

There is always one moment in childhood when the door opens and lets the future in.

****

Comment 3

To be grown up is to slowly forget the things you wondered about as a child.

****

Comment 4

Childhood is the world of miracle or of magic: it is as if creation rose luminously out of the night, all new and fresh and astonishing.

Task A: Essay Sample 37
Comment Set V

It is true that childhood is the world of magic or miracle as anything seems possible due to less stresses of everyday life. However only some are able to experience this magic as some childhoods are stripped away due to the unpleasant circumstances like child labor as a result of poor economic state of a nation. This can have several poor consequences which are worth investigating.

Childhood is the world of magic however some childhood experiences are not magical due to child labor. Normally, childhood is considered magical when a child is able to connect, talk, play and live in a healthy home and community. According to some studies 90% of a child's brain is developed by the age of 5. Hence, it is important to inculcate these five things early in life to increase creativity and growth mindset which has several benefits as an adult. However, this notion is challenged by certain structures in the society that lead to circumstances where an individual is unable to experience that magic. Normally, the resources and the economic situation of a nation decide the fate of a childhood. For example, kids in developing nations like Afghanistan would never be able to experience a magical childhood when compared to kids in Australia. Since Afghanistan is undergoing economic crisis and poverty, families can't even afford the basic necessities of life. In such circumstances, some children are forced to do child labor which can be a traumatic experience. Due to the increased stresses early in life these children never get to experience a world where everything is magical and possible. When these children grow up with these traumatic experiences, they experience mental health disorders and can never compete with children of their age from developed nations. Hence, the economic situation of a nation can decide whether a childhood would be magical or not.

To counter the problems of child labor, ideally we would want all the nations to be economically stable and free of poverty. However this prospect is difficult to achieve in a short span of time. Hence, we could enforce ban on the products made by children in developing nations. However a complete ban would mean that they don't have any source of income which is not practical. This can force the children and adults to resort to underground jobs like prostitution which can be even more traumatic. Hence, developing nations can adopt others measures that are practical such as poor working conditions should be strictly forbidden, working hours should be limited and the nature of tasks should be corresponding with the physical and mental abilities of the children performing them. Furthermore, firms employing children should offer prospects for improvement, such as offering on-site schooling after work. This solution will solve the problem of poverty as well as the barriers to education.

Childhood is a beautiful experience and every child should have the right to experience that to the fullest. However there are certain structures in the society such as the economic state of a nation that can decide the fate of a childhood. Lack of resources and poor job opportunities can lead to poverty which can lead to traumatic childhood experiences like child labor. In order to counter this problem it is vital for the employers to ensure that the working conditions for children are safe and also onsite education is provided after work.

Comment Set W

Comment 1

The internet is so big, so powerful and pointless that for some people it is a complete substitute for life

****

Comment 2

For a successful technology, reality must take precedence over public relations, for Nature cannot be fooled

****

Comment 3

Humanity is acquiring all the right technology for all the wrong reasons

****

Comment 4

The new electronic independent re-creates the image of a global village

Task A: Essay Sample 38
Comment Set W

It is true that technology is a powerful commodity in 21 st century. It has many advantages like it aids in quick communication, spreading a positive message or marketing which can boost the economy. However, technology is feeding on us instead of us feeding on the technology which is concerning. Social media such as instagram, snapchat or facebook are examples of digital technology that we have been abusing since its inception. This technology has advantages only when used in balance or else it can be that powerful monster that can consume an individual and obscure their sense of reality. This sense of reality is a key to happy and fulfilling life which has a meaning and purpose.

In today's world, digital technology can prove to obscure our reality when not used in an appropriate manner. Social media like instagram is an example of digital media which has gained popularity in a short span of time. This platform has obscured our reality and made us culprits of our own limited freedom. We control our public relation by creating an image of ourselves on social media. This image could not be a reality of us but we still do it to please other people and to fit in to the society. Humans have always had the instinct to fit in and in order to achieve that we follow what other people are doing. We are essentially compromising our authenticity for instant gratification. We get happy when someone likes, comments or shares our posts. We don't realize that these posts are gimmicks that release dopamine which gives us instant gratification. This happiness is not sustainable and it can never replace true compliments that we can give each other when we are face to face. Furthermore, according to some studies, it has been found that children that spend more time on their phone had less developed frontal cortex. It is a vital issue as frontal cortex plays an important role in rational decision making. Hence, it is upto us how we want to make use of the technology.

To counter this, we need to learn to maintain a balance between social media and our life. One could go complete turkey if one can't maintain a balance or one could realize the negatives of social media and maintain a balance and only use it to our advantage. One could use it for marketing a specific product to expand business or for the welfare of the society by spreading a positive message. For example some people have pages on instagram where they market their products like crochets. People can visit these pages and order a crochet. It is a quick and hassle free selling and buying of products. Either going complete turkey or maintaining a balance, both will lead to a path that will promote freedom to be with oneself. Balance can be achieved by limiting the time spent on social media, not comparing oneself to other people, not seeking gratification when someone likes posts and putting other main roles of our life first like spending time with family and with oneself. This freedom to be with oneself is a key to a fulfilling life. One can reach our full potential only when an individual has a true sense of purpose and meaning in life which can be achieved when our reality is not obscured by factors like digital technology. Hence it is important to identify how the technology is adding value to one's life and when it is obscuring the reality. After determining that, one can take appropriate action to control our behaviors.

Social media is an example of digital technology which has both positives and negatives. It can prove to be detrimental when not used in an appropriate manner. Hence, it is important to find that right balance otherwise we are at a risk of living a life that is not fulfilling and authentic.

Comment Set X

Comment 1

Farms-scale trial plots of genetically modified crops are rather like letting a rat with bubonic plague out into the environment and then seeing what happens.

Patrick Holden

****

Comment 2

Someday a child is going to sue its parents for being born. They will say, my life is so awful with these terrible genetic defects and you just callously didn't find out.

James D. Watson.

Comment 3

Genetic control will be the weapon of the future.

Jeanette Winterson

****

Comment 4

Life is a copiously branching bush, continually pruned by the grim reaper of unsuitability and extinction, not a ladder of predictable progress.

Stephen Jay Gould

Task A: Essay Sample 39
Comment Set X

Title 1: Genes for Genes

Title 2: "Hey, Those are Some Nice Genes you're Wearing!"

Title 3: "Hey, Nice Genes!"

Who does not want their child to be disease and defect free? For that matter, what child does not wish to have been born with all their defects and allergies? Surely, if any parent had the chance to make this happen safely they would take the chance. However, it is this very issue of safety that is key. So much uncertainty yet surrounds this new field. In addition, worries abound that research and experience in this field will be transferred to unrelated and more harmful industries. As such, although genetic control and modification have their benefits, it may be best to leave things as they are.

Genetic selection and modification can have their benefits. The various diseases and defects that people are born with, and which cost the healthcare system billions of dollars a year to treat, make this new science a tempting area to explore and develop further. Apart from the medical costs, there are also the inconveniences that children have to live with. For example, if a child was born without sight or without a limb, it would make life very difficult for them in this tough world. Indeed, they may even be inclined to sue their parents for such inconveniences they have to live with, as Watson alluded to. Furthermore, why stop at just preventing diseases? If it were possible to make someone taller, smarter, and stronger, why not pursue this too? As such, genetic engineering seems like a good and beneficial area to pursue.

However, the safety and uncertainty concerns are such that it would be best to let things be natural. This is yet an emerging science with little to no longer-term trials having taken place with live human subjects. The uncertainties, and dangers, abound. Indeed, the Thalidomide scandal from a few decades ago, where babies were born with severe defects, demonstrates the dangers of administering unfamiliar medical treatments on live human subjects. As Holden was alluding to, scientists may be unleashing something horrendous that is yet to be comprehended. What is more, even if all goes as planned, and diseases are treated well, who knows what else such genetic manipulation will be used for. Time and time again, it has been observed how science has been turned towards military uses. An example was Einstein's research into the power of the splitting of the atom. Indeed, such genetic modification may be used to create 'super soldiers' - human beings with superhuman strength to go to war against other countries. Thus, an arms race will ensue in genetic modification and it will get out of hand, such that those who are not genetically modified will feel like inferior human beings. As such, it would be better if scientists and citizens just let their own genetics run their natural course. There are too many uncertainties for both safety and the wonton inclinations of mankind.

In conclusion, although there are benefits to genetic engineering, it would be better if humankind let their genes alone. The benefits of genetic medication may erase diseases in children before they are born, thus saving a lot of cost and inconvenience. Furthermore, such science may be used to create 'improved' human beings. Despite this, there remains plenty of uncertainty and risk. More harm may be done to children in this new science. Furthermore, genetic modification may be abused to create people with superhuman abilities, potentially unleashing a greater menace upon humankind.

Comment Set Y

Comment 1

What is lawful and what is just are not the same thing.

****

Comment 2

Legal systems are an essential element of democracies.

****

Comment 3

Behind every great fortune there is crime.

****

Comment 4

Society prepares the crime; the criminal commits it.

Task A: Essay Sample 40
Comment Set Y

The dominant narrative of Australian society compels many to believe that our legal system is just. However, unfair and oppressive behaviours occur within society with the sanction of the law. Furthermore, the same laws may be applied differently for different people. As such, even though people are made to believe that the legal system is just, the reality is that it allows injustices to abound.

We are made to believe that our legal system is just. This is to say, the bad are punished and the good are upheld. To ensure this, we are told the police and the courts exist. Although not everyone has personal experience with these institutions, we have a feeling that they will be 'on our side' if ever we find ourselves in a dispute or altercation and we know that we had done nothing wrong. Where do these feelings come from? They may arise from our youth from watching television shows and movies where law enforcement are portrayed as heroes who make sure that good prevails. Such feelings may also arise from watching newscasters and politicians on television constantly asserting to us that we live in a liberal democracy, of which the legal system is an essential element. This is the 'superstructure' of our society, according to Marx. That is to say, these are the controlling images that form part of the dominant narrative of what society is. As such, it can be seen how many people would be led to believe that our legal system in Australia is just.

However, the reality is that injustice abounds in our legal system. This can be seen with both the law itself and also the unfair application of it. Regarding the law, injustice can be seen with how it protects the rights and interests of those who currently hold power. For example, this may be seen with landlords who insist on full rent and who evict renters who are struggling during this pandemic. Some of these renters had to dip into their savings and superannuation to help pay this rent. In effect, there has been a wealth transfer during this pandemic where the rich got richer, and the poor, poorer. However, under the legal system in Australia, the landlord has free reign to charge as they please and to evict these renters. Although the government imposed a brief moratorium, that has now passed. As such, what the landlords are doing is completely legal under the law, but it is not just. In traditional Indigenous society in Australia, the law of 'usufruct' was the norm. That is to say, property and food was distributed and shared on a needs basis. Indeed, human life and well-being was sacrosanct under Indigenous laws. However, under modern Australian law, 'property' rights are now treated as sacrosanct. This is ironic given that it was the contravention of the common law property rights of Aboriginal peoples (which the Mabo Case affirmed the Crown was meant to respect), and the various other crimes the colonialists perpetuated against them in the Frontier Wars, which led to the land holdings and good fortune of most Australians at present. Similar unfair applications of the law can be observed in the present. For example, it can be observed how the Australian legal system arrests and jails Aboriginal peoples at a proportion much greater than their populational representation. An example of this was

Tanya Day whom the Victorian police arrested and put into a police cell for merely being drunk in public and not hurting anyone. She was subsequently left to die in a prison cell whilst being medically unattended. If Tanya Day was Caucasian, the police would probably have just given her a verbal reprimand and told to go home, or else even driven her home themselves. Another unfair application of modern Australian law can be seen with the very low conviction rate of perpetrators of sexual assault against women. As such, injustice abounds in our current legal system, both with the laws them self and with how the legal system applies them.

In conclusion, even though we are made to believe that our legal system in Australia is just, it is really full of injustice, both in the substance of the law and in its application. The dominant narrative in society, instilled through popular culture and politicians, portrays the idea that the Australian legal system is just. However, an examination of the landlord-renter relationship, and of the treatment of Aboriginal peoples, both past and present, reveals how the legal system in Australia allows injustices to abound.

Looking for more? No problemo! More sample, model essays can be found online in your gamsat-prep.com account.

5.1.2 Writing Task B Model Essays

Comment Set A

Comment 1

A man's growth is seen in the successive choirs of his friends.

Ralph Waldo Emerson

****

Comment 2

Friendship is a single soul dwelling in two bodies.

Aristotle

****

Comment 3

I have friends in overalls whose friendship I would not swap for the favor of the kings of the world.

Thomas Edison

****

Comment 4

The bird a nest, the spider a web, man friendship.

William Blake

Task B: Essay Sample 1
Comment Set A

Ar Scath a Chéile Maireann na Daoine.

Friendship is a miracle. Some friendships are different to others, some are lifelong, some are unexpected, some are fleeting. Friends always have our best interests and we can rely on them to provide joy, support, honesty and often a shoulder to cry on.

One of my best friends, Raidin, I met in college, we had the same sort of upbringing, and our parents, on the few occasions they met got on like a house on fire. When Raidin's mum became very ill, she went home for a few weeks to be with her mum, my friends and I missed her terribly, she was (and still is) the life and soul of the party! Our house was so quiet without her playing goofy music or dancing around.

We were starting a new module about writing our thesis and it was very complicated, Raidin, unfortunately, missed the first few weeks and since the module was delivered in face-to-face tutorials I knew she would struggle to keep up with what was going on. We were in contact with her on the group chat every day and my friends and I took it upon ourselves to approach the lecturer after the second tutorial to make a special request. We explained the situation, emphasising how Raidin lived two hours away from UCD and how ill her mum was and asked her if there was any way she would be able to facilitate a special one on one tutorial on facetime. She was so thankful that it had been brought to her attention as obviously our thesis would count towards our final score. She conducted the tutorial on facetime so Raidin could remain at home caring for her mum and still not be overwhelmed by the workload when she returned to Dublin.

Raidin's mum passed away shortly after that. She was distraught and needed all of the support we could give. Things were spiralling out of control, on nights out she would drink excessively to forget the trauma of the months before, she was neglecting her college work and slipping further and further behind. One Sunday night when we were all back in the house after the weekend with our families, we made an intervention, we told her it was okay to feel so terrible, she had just been robbed of one of the most important and influential people in her life. We said acting in such a destructive manner was not going to help the situation. She didn't need to pretend she was okay, we made it clear she could speak to us about anything and that if she wanted to apply for extensions and accommodations on her assignments, we would help her.

Part of being a good friend is supporting and helping each other through difficult times and being honest with each other, however harsh or painful the truth may be. After that long talk with Raidin ,things improved, we helped her apply for extensions and every one was granted, she got through the year achieving a 1:1 degree. I can't imagine there could have been anyone prouder than her mum.

Friendship is one of the foundations upon which society is built, everyone needs a friend from time to time regardless of who they are or what status they bear. Without friends we become introverted and lonely, think of the importance of the friends elderly people have in day-care centres or the friends children have in school. Think of how much they have missed those friends during the lockdown due to Covid-19. The measures people went to keep in contact with their friends during the restrictions, for instance, chatting over garden walls or on facetime is a testimony of the importance of friends for love and support, as said by Aristotle, 'friendship is a single soul dwelling in two bodies'.

To conclude, good friends make us better people, we can trust them to watch out of us, be honest with us and they always have our best interests at heart. We need them like an animal needs shelter, as said by William Blake, 'The bird a nest, the spider a web, man friendship', with true friends we will always be at home. As the old Irish saying goes, 'ar scath a chéile, maireann na daoine', under the shelter of others people survive.

Task B: Essay Sample 2
Comment Set A

I lifted my phone in front of my face and tried to focus my eyes on the time. This task was not helped by the fact that I didn't have my glasses on. And the fact that I was incredibly drunk.

Almost 5am. Christ. I put my phone down and looked around the room. My friends were sprawled across the two couches in our sitting room, perched at a variety of interesting, even artistic, angles. Some toe-to-toe with others, some sprawled over the side, one even upside down.

The only other person awake was Ciara. It had been a late one. While most of our friends that night had been drinking to have a good time, I was drowning my sorrows. My first proper relationship had just come to an end after two years, ending over the phone. I wanted to forget, and now Ciara and I were the last two standing (sitting), taking turns to swing from a bottle of wine.

Ciara was one of the few I had trusted to tell. She and her boyfriend of four years had broken up several months ago. While there was no big fight, more simply two people moving in different directions, she was devastated nonetheless.

As I lolled about, trying to remain conscious and wallowing in a mixture of sadness and self-pity, I worked up the courage to ask: "So this is what it feels like?"

"Yes". She didn't say anything else. She didn't have to, and just that knowledge that she knew exactly what I was going through was enough for me.

I'm not sure if I had realised before that point just how crucial a part of my life my friends really were. For most of my life, friends had been someone to play Playstation with, another body there for football.

My drunken pity-party two years after finishing college was one of first times it clicked what friendship really meant. That support on offer, impossible for someone who doesn't know you or who you don't like to give. That feeling of a true bond, with someone who is family in all but name. A real and genuine love - not romantic or familial, but one that is just as strong and important nonetheless.

When I looked back, I realised my friends had played a massive part in my life even before that. Theresa, a friend a few years older than me in college, encouraging me to move in with her and some other mates when I was just 20 and had never lived out of home. The daily phone calls with Liam during my Leaving Cert exams, talking incredibly value nonsense that helped to keep me sane.

While there is plenty good, there are of course lots of potential downsides from friendships. The fights and bust ups. Or, often more painful, the person you once thought a brother slowly drifting out of your life due to bad luck, a change of location, indifference, or one of a million reasons.

Like any relationship, where there is the potential for joy, there is the potential for pain. But for most, the scale will be tipped very strongly in favour of the light. For most, your friends will be the ones to lift you up when you fall. Or lie on the ground with you when you're drunk and miserable. Both are equally important.

Comment Set B

Comment 1

The worst loneliness is not to be comfortable with yourself.

Mark Twain

****

Comment 2

Solitude is the profoundest fact of the human condition. Man is the only being who knows he is alone.

Octavio Paz

****

Comment 3

Loneliness is a barrier that prevents one from uniting with the inner self.

Carl Rogers

****

Comment 4

At the innermost core of all loneliness is a deep and powerful yearning for union with one's lost self.

Brendan Francis

Task B: Essay Sample 3
Comment Set B

"Loneliness is a barrier that prevents on from reuniting with their inner self"

Mankind are innately social creatures. Social interaction is the medium for a healthy exchange of ideas, may serve as a catharsis for inner turmoil, and is essential for support and to form genuine companionships. Thus, one of the most debilitating fears of mankind is loneliness; the feeling of distress and hopelessness when being alone and devoid of companionship, or even the sensation of feeling disconnected from the world around you. People feel as though it is "them against the world." However, I believe that nobody is ever truly lonely if learn to cherish solitude and nurture their inner self. Carl Rogers' quote "loneliness is a barrier that prevents on from reuniting with their inner self" expresses that loneliness is merely a state of mind and that happiness can be found when relinquishing this perception and reconciling with our inner self.

My transition from high school to university was imbued with the fervent expectations of establishing a close group of friends that I would retain throughout adulthood. Forming friendships in high school was easy because the constant contact with the same peers and history of memories and growing up together forged solid connections. However, university life thrust me into a whole new dimension and my expectations were shattered. The immense population of university and the multitude of different classes rendered it difficult to keep contact with others and students were well aware of the impermanence of passing social interaction, thereby deciding to withdraw. I found myself drowning in an ocean of indifference; a hectic schedule full of lecture halls where students neglected the presence of those around them, tutorials with students only exchanging names then ceasing social interactions, wandering along a main walkway surrounded by so many people but not knowing a soul around me. Needless to say, I felt very lonely.

With the advent of social media, I felt increasingly pressured to socialise or even project an illusion of happiness by attending social events. Plagued by peer pressure, I attended a few university events in the hope of fulfilling the typical "uni student mould," but was left utterly disillusioned. It seemed that students preferred to take advantage of the open bar rather than engage in meaningful conversations. The mindless "small talk" I had to feign interest in gave rise to a nagging sense of emptiness within me. Feeling unfulfilled by the experience and alienated, I felt lonely in a crowded room.

One day to clear up my inner turmoil, I took a solitary hike in Royal National Park. Somehow this time, my eye caught certain details I never noticed before; iridescent threads of colour on every leaf, the unique tonality of bird calls and even the intricate patterns etched into the bark of an oak tree. I marvelled at the majesty of the tree and found its antiquity unfathomable. I wondered how much this tree has seen in its lifetime, how many handprints its bark bore, how many people its encountered. Somehow, I felt inexplicable security its antiquity and wisdom which had endured the test of time. Venturing on, I let the dizzying cliffs overlooking the wide expanse of sea engulf me completely. It was incredible sensation, feeling tiny in a ginormous world; a sensation which trivialised my worries and cares. This brief escape left me truly refreshed, and I regained my strength and motivation to face the world again.

I derived my strength and energy from enjoying the tranquillity of nature and nurturing a rich inner world; all the markings of an introvert. However, I decided to embrace this realisation. My initial perceived loneliness and inadequacy of not being able to connect sufficiently with others was only interpreted through the lens of social expectations, namely into what an adolescent was meant to embrace. It took me quite a while to realise everyone's lives was propelled by their autonomy; as soon as I relinquished my feelings of loneliness, I became more comfortable in my own skin. I decided to nurture my inner self by immersing myself in stories- I was able to traverse distant lands vicariously through Bilbo Baggins, Harry Potter, Elizabeth Bennett. I embraced the therapeutic simplicity of origami, attempted to cook and even picked up French again. I was the happiest when I listened to myself, when I experienced growth and learnt new skills. In addition, I even ventured to join a few social clubs at uni, such as a taekwondo club where I made friends with those with similar interests to me.

Loneliness is a debilitating state of mind defined by the complete loss of hope in companionship anywhere. However, it is undeniable that there is still strength within oneself, and the infinite capacity to seek happiness within; it is our responsibility to judge how we feel and indulge in fulfilling pursuits. Nobody is ever truly lonely, as loneliness is only a state of mind, a barrier which can only be surmounted once we reconcile with and embrace our inner self.

Task B: Essay Sample 4
Comment Set B

Me

21 April, 2012. 7:32 pm. Screech. Crash. The sound of the impact deafening. Ringing in my ears. Blood trickling down my cheekbone. The grasp of the seatbelt tight around my waist. I look left. I see her. Her body motionless. Her face peaceful. Gone.

Two years on from this accident and I am standing at the start of the Nullarbor. Or was it the end? A 260km asphalt line on the surface of the earth running out to the horizon. Dead straight. This felt like a physical representation of my life since that April night two years ago. The only difference was this was above the surface, my internal road felt like it was along the depth pit of Hell.

Today, I can look back on my experiences from a nicer place. A location with a view over the ocean, the waves gently rolling in onto the golden sands. To me this is a place of inner peace, of meaningful relationships, of self-contentment.

After the accident, I went through the typical stages of grief. Denial, anger, sadness. My inability to express feelings and emotions made this a difficult period for everyone around me. It eventually resulted in the loss of all friendship. When I felt like I needed everyone the most, I was at a point of abandonment. I was physical present in society. Attended work, presented my body to family events but my mind was absent. Something inside of me also passed away that fateful night in April. I did not like who I was becoming. But also had no control over the downward spiral that was my once promising life. Mark Twain reflects the way I was feeling. "The worst loneliness is not to be comfortable with yourself". I agree with this wholeheartedly. I could not even stand to be around myself. How I was going to tolerate life at this point? This is not how I envisaged my life was going to turn out. Alone. Desolate. Desperate. Despair.

Standing at the start of that road two years later was the most important and symbolic moment in my life. I had to go back. I had to face the demons of the past life. I knew that driving along this stretch of seemingly endless highway would be tough. It was going to mark the resurrection of my soul. A new chapter in my life. And I felt compelled to do it alone. After all, I did not have much left back at home. It was from this moment I needed to find out about myself. Who was I at the root element? What was my purpose? I was alone.

"To dare to live alone is the rarest courage; since there are many who had rather meet their bitterest enemy in the field, than their own hearts in their closet" (Charles Caleb Colton). I was alone. Isolated. No human companionship. No friendship with anything. I had no choice but to meet my own heart. Face my own fears. To reignite the light, I drove by day, I drove by night, experiencing the wilderness of the outback. I felt like Matthew Flinders circumnavigating Australia for the first time. Thriving in the isolation. I met many people along the way. Some like me, others very different. There was no judgment, no prejudice. Just true human experience, human connection. I forced myself to open my heart. I reflected back on my life whilst undertaking this journey of self-discovery. Self-fulfilment. It was a journey planned by two people, and walked by one.

I sit here now, reflecting back on my life. Since I am unable to change the events of that night, I cannot but accept the outcome. But I am grateful for the journey of isolation and loneliness that I have experienced since then. I was a lost sheep, walking amongst a blurred flock. I found myself yearning for connection, yet did not know how to grasp it. The Shepard in my heart, in my soul, led me through the darkness and into the light of today. Today, rich with connection, spoilt with emotion and most importantly, with love of myself. I am me.

Task B: Essay Sample 5
Comment Set B

"The worst loneliness is not to be comfortable with yourself."

Until this year, I would not have been able to say whether I agreed or disagreed with Mark Twain on the above statement. I had never been truly lonely, and so had never been forced to confront myself. Recent circumstances have changed this.

I came to Australia on a 6-month sabbatical from an easy, well-paid but mindless job in Ireland. The plan was to spend my time doing casual work, travelling and partying. Then back to Ireland and my comfortable drudgery.

Well, men make plans and God laughs. The economic effects of Covid-19 meant that my job at home suddenly no longer existed. Furthermore, because I wasn't technically employed in Ireland when the so-called pandemic payments were allotted, I would have had no source of income whatsoever should I have decided to return. I was in a quandary. What made things worse is that casual labouring work in Sydney dried up with the advent of lockdown. All at once, I was unemployed and with rapidly-dwindling resources.

A phone call from a friend saved me. The company he worked for had won a contract down on the south coast to clean up the remnants of houses that had been burned out by the bush fires. Free food and board, decent pay, the opportunity to see the countryside. It was exactly what I needed.

However, I failed to account for one thing. I was assailed by crippling loneliness almost from the first day. Although my friend and I were sharing a house, his position as site manager meant that he was often out and about, leaving me with only myself for company. For someone who has always been a social animal, it was an enormous struggle. I felt isolated and utterly alone. It seemed that I was carrying a huge weight around in my belly from the moment I awoke in the morning to when I finally drifted into the sleep I so craved at night.

Thankfully, some good came of it. My seemingly endless hours alone caused some real introspection. I examined my life up to that point. I realised that I hadn't felt fulfilled or truly happy in years. It became obvious to me that I had been sleepwalking through my life since I left school, simply taking whatever opportunities arose and allowing others to shape my path. I asked myself what I really wanted. The answer was, to take agency of myself. To forge a career that I could be proud of. To push myself to achieve what I believe myself to be capable of. I decided I was going to become a doctor.

As soon as the thought arrived fully-formed in my head, I knew it was the right decision. The obstacles in my way, exams, cost, time, only served to heighten my determination. A new sense of purpose came over me, so that everything I have done form then on has been to that end.

This could never have happened without the enforced loneliness I had to endure. It taught me so much, though. Most of all, that to be uncomfortable with yourself may be a curse, but it is one you can break, if you truly want to.

Comment Set C

Comment 1

Courage is a mean with regard to fear and confidence.

Aristotle

****

Comment 2

Courage is of the heart by derivation,
And great it is. But fear is of the soul.

Robert Frost

****

Comment 3

Courage doesn't always roar. Sometimes courage is the little voice at the end of the day that says I'll try again tomorrow.

Mary Anne Radmacher

****

Comment 4

Courage is being scared to death— and saddling up anyway.

John Wayne

Task B: Essay Sample 6
Comment Set C

To my child,

Today you see me sitting in this beautiful office that overlooks the hospital on one side and the view of the River Torrens on the other. You see my accomplishments lined across the walls, my certificates, my degrees and our family photos. I see your face when you see these things, you ask questions but I see you in mesmerised by all these achievements.

You were only born 13 years ago, and my daughter they have been the best 13 years. I am writing you this letter because I want you to know that the years before that and even the years you have been alive, life hasn't always been rainbows and sunshine. I was a young girl who was always told I could achieve anything I set my mind to, but that wasn't always that case. I finished year 12 with marks that still shock me for all the wrong reasons. I was lying in a bed in Paris and I just about soaked a pillow with my tears. I worked hard, I had tutors, I never went out and still I wasn't in the top 10% of the state. I was crushed. I would wake up every morning after that and think, can I even become a doctor? Is there any point trying anymore? I remember finally leaving the hotel room and walking around, for some reason I kept finding myself circulating the medical school. I looked up at that building and thought, I am not giving up. This is not the end.

Then I researched all my possible options, could I re-do the year from hell? Could I start a degree that would help me do postgraduate medicine? As you know I went with the later, but again it was not easy. I studied for 3 years with the intention that I would get straight in, not realising that there was the devil, the GAMSAT exam that would get in my way. I still remember the feeling of opening my results and thinking, THIS IS IT! Third time lucky, I've done it. All to realise in later months that I missed out on an interview by one point. I was transferred back to that feeling in Paris, the feeling of worthlessness. I had given up hope. I started considering other options, maybe I could just follow in my mother's footsteps, maybe I could be an accountant after all. I pondered the idea, but it did not make me happy. I thought about all the mundane things in my life and my career was not going to be one of them.

The words of aunties and friends would taunt me "why don't you just do something else? How much longer are you going to chase this ridiculous dream? How much money are you going to spend doing this?" This was the thing that caused me to spiral. But it became my encouragement, not only was I doing this for myself but I was doing this to prove them all wrong. The little voice in my head said just give it one more shot.

So again, I started studying this was my third summer of not going out an being locked in my room, facing 1000s of questions again. I am so thankful that I shut out all the hatred that year, because that little voice was right. 2018 was my year. I did get accepted.

I wanted to write this down for you, so that on days that are tough you have a reason to keep trying, a reason to be strong. Although, right now it seems like I have it all, there is a time where I was convinced that my life would amount to nothing. Every time someone puts you down, I want you to remember that little voice inside your head, that voice is one of the most powerful things especially when it is filled with hope and courage. Courage is knowing that sometimes your decision isn't going to be favoured, but believing in yourself enough not to listen to these critics.

YOU ARE STRONG, YOU CAN ACHIEVE ANYTHING!

Love you,

Mum x

Comment Set D

Comment 1

In the end, everything is a gag.

Charlie Chaplin

Task B: Essay Sample 7
Comment Set D

What is so funny?

"In the end, everything is a gag." These profound words, uttered by Charlie Chaplin, one of the earliest comedians of the 20th century, speak a myriad of truth about the double-edged nature of humour. Sadly, on our current culture, even the most sensitive subjects are not safe from ridicule and parody. As a young adult growing in this often cruel society, I am often questioning the extent of what we consider to be humorous. Taken in the same frame of mind as Charlie Chaplin's words, if something can be made fun of, then it will eventually be ridiculed. This extreme line of thought left an uneasy impression on me when I least expected it.

For a greater part of my childhood, I have been an avid fan of the cartoon show, South Park. South Park is well known for its risqué and offensive parody type of humour. In one particular episode, the show satirised the sensitive issue of AIDS. Despite laughing at its comical moments, that specific episode left a disturbing afterthought. Would I have found that type of humour entertaining if I was afflicted with the deadly AIDS disease? This led to the other questions of why the general population sees this as acceptable humour. Decades ago, during the initial outbreak of AIDS, such humour would have caused outrage nationwide and led to the cancellation of South Park. However, in today's society, it barely caused a ripple. It seems that all issues in our contemporary world are being sucked into a vortex of no-limits all out comedy, and people don't seem to care as much as before.

Similarly, the show 'Chaser's War on Everything' did a parody sketch on real terminally ill children. This epitomises the idea that nothing is safe from ridicule and parody. Children on their death beds, being ridiculed on national television! Comedy has evolved in great magnitudes since the days of Charlie Chaplin. But even then, Chaplin rightly predicted that eventually, all issues can and will be subject to satire.

I have come to realise that even though nothing is safe from ridicule, we must keep an open mind on what as an acceptable for of comedy. Though it may be hilarious to one person, we must empathise with those being ridiculed. It will only be a matter of time before something close to your heart will be taken by the growing 'black hole of comedy'.

Comment Set E

Comment 1

In every man's heart there is a secret nerve that answers to the vibrations of beauty.

Christopher Morley

****

Comment 2

I see beauty as the grace point between what hurts and what heals, between the shadow of tragedy and the light of joy. I find beauty in my scars.

****

Comment 3

What makes the desert beautiful is that somewhere it hides a well.

The Little Prince, Antoine de Saint Exupery

****

Comment 4

When you have only two pennies left in the world, buy a loaf of bread with one, and a lily with the other.

Chinese Proverb

Task B: Essay Sample 8
Comment Set E

Beauty is invisible to the eye

I read the Little Prince when I was young and I never fully understood the concept of hidden beauty until I was I high school. Growing up, I would always be bombarded with magazines and magazine that depict flawless models and place importance on external looks. In today's society, not much importance is given to building one's character and every individual is adamant on looking good on the outside. The perverse notion of outer beauty has gone to such an extent that people are undergoing surgery to obtain the perfectly chiselled jawline of Brad Pitt or the sculpted rear of Jennifer Lopez.

During my high school days, I relished on the attention that I received from boys my age. They thought I was beautiful and I loved being beautiful. I placed a great deal of importance, energy, and money in the way I looked on the outside. I bought expensive make-up products, booked monthly salon appointments for my highly coloured and extension-ridden hair. However, I paid little importance to who I was becoming on the inside. Being popular was my forte and I excelled at it. All of that changed when I noticed my hair falling out in the shower. I had a patch of my scalp that was visible. When I went to see the dermatologist, I was diagnosed with Alopecia.

Within months, I had lost all my hair and this greatly impacted my emotional well-being and self-esteem. Going to a high school in which the students place importance on one's outer appearance, it was a hard downfall from being the popular student in school to becoming someone who was completely bald. When my boyfriend ended our relationship because of my condition, I realised that outer beauty is just a façade, a mask, for your inner self. I found strength in the knowledge that my outer appearance is not a representation of who I am on the inside. I started joining more clubs and societies in school and met amazing and like-minded individuals who did not rate someone based on their appearance but on their character. Learning the hidden treasures of someone's true character that is concealed by their outward mask was an important life lesson for me.

Not many people in today's society realise that beauty is just a transient mask. What lies underneath is the true representation of a person. A person's beauty can be withered into nothingness due to old age but the character of a person stands true through time. There have been countless cases in which young girls are so obsessed with looking beautiful like the actresses and singers on television that they surgically change their appearance. What they do not realise is the extent of the prevalence of Photoshop in the industry. A societal change needs to be undergone to educate the people about the crucial nature of developing one personality rather than beauty. Personality cannot go through liposuction for enhancement, it needs to be cultivated. Singers and actors should set an example as role models for the younger generations by promoting inner beauty instead of focusing solely on the outer. After all, maybe the next unappealing person you meet in the future could be the nicest and most helpful individual that you have ever come across.

Task B: Essay Sample 9
Comment Set E

When will we be beautiful?

Beauty goes beyond skin deep. This is the way we teach children to perceive the world. Homo sapiens have the highest degree of cognitive ability throughout the animal kingdom. The fact that we are aware makes it our duty to reason and moralise. As such, it has become our inherent nature to differentiate between good actions and bad actions. A philosopher resides within us all. The philosopher within Antoine de Saint-Exupery said, "What makes the desert beautiful is that somewhere it hides a well."

While we do our best to impart moral values onto new generations, we can also observe that it is not within the nature of the human race to be prejudiced. Prejudice usually comes from the teachings of others or out of instincts to be wary of our differences. So why then, is it still necessary to teach moral values? It could be possible that without guidance, people would naturally attain the outlook we would aim for anyway. I was taught moral values as a child. Although my family had a religion, we weren't always very good at practising it, However, moral values and religious values are one and the same, and so they superseded religious rituals.

When I was nine, I moved to a new school and was almost immediately befriended by a girl in my class who suffered from cerebral palsy. She didn't have many friends because it seemed that the other students quickly grew tired of her. Everyone had trouble understanding her when she spoke because of her partial paralysis, as she wasn't as physically able as the rest of us. I immediately thought everyone was terrible shallow for not having patience with her until I found out that I was also strained from my companionship with her. It felt like a real struggle being slowed down all the time. I was her only friend and I was finding it difficult. I knew that beauty went beyond skin deep but that didn't seem to make it any easier. Upon reflection now. Many years later, I realise that people are not immoral. They simply struggle between whether to put themselves first or to put others with greater needs first.

It is necessary to teach oral values but it is infinitely more necessary to us to realise them. Everyone is an individual within a community. Most people have opinions. Some express those opinions. Everyone is trying to achieve the right outcome, but do we truly realise our morals? Until it becomes our goal to find the well in the desert, the inner beauty we all have, we will always be putting ourselves before others.

Comment Set F

Comment 1

Experience is not what happens to you. It is what you do with what happens to you.

****

Comment 2

It is not only for what we do that we are held responsible, but also for what we do not do.

****

Comment 3

Experience is a hard teacher because she gives the test first, the lesson afterward.

****

Comment 4

Life teaches none but those who study it.

Task B: Essay Sample 10
Comment Set F

Every day is a new experience, many of us would love to think we have never made a mistake big enough to have impacted on our whole lives, I myself didn't think I had until I took some time to reflect before writing this essay. Our mistakes are our number one teacher but it is detrimental to let mistakes happen and not learn from them, it is from these mistakes that we can improve ourselves and make better, more positive decisions in the future.

Life is the best teacher. For as long as I can remember I have wanted to study medicine, I aimed for it the whole way through secondary school, spending evenings watching Greys Anatomy and New Amsterdam, I am aware that these are not full representations of a doctor's job but their ability to help people and the buzz they got from it amazed me. I sat the HPAT exam and did better than I would have thought, however I struggled with languages in school such as French and Irish, I didn't have an interest in them and knew that in medicine I wouldn't need them as much as I would maths and science. As a result of this I didn't score highly enough in my leaving certificate to get offered a place in any of the undergraduate medicine courses. I was only 16 when I sat the leaving cert so I decided I would sit it again the following year, I studied a lot harder but, alas, I just missed out. I wallowed for days and eventually decided against advice not to do it a third time and accepted a place on a nursing course in UCD. My confidence was shattered and I didn't want to go through the heartbreak of missing out on a spot in the course a third time.

I studied nursing, I enjoyed some placements more than others, I quickly learned that I liked acute settings and when I qualified, I accepted a job in an oncology ward. Medicine was still on my mind, it was my dream, but I didn't have the courage to pursue it further. I loved the clinical side of nursing but the day-to-day work was quickly becoming monotonous and boring. I yearned for more. I made a list of everything I enjoyed about looking after patients, I loved the social side, I loved when they came in to the hospital ill and there was a puzzle to be solved re finding out what was causing their problems. I loved the monitoring of ill patients and seeing them improve day by day. The idea of studying medicine came, once again to the forefront.

My big mistake I quickly realised that I had let myself stop learning, I let myself get too comfortable in my job that I supressed my ambition to study medicine. There was no one to blame but myself, I had failed myself by not pursuing my dream and taking the easy way out. I struggled with this and felt ever so cowardly. I had to take responsibility for myself and registered to sit the GAMSAT in the hope of studying post-graduate medicine.

Fortunately, I was able to identify my mistake and am doing all I possibly can to rectify it before it is too late. In society many people have regrets, they regret failed relationships, not pursuing their careers, not saving more money or not spending enough time with their families. I have learned with experience that one must aggressively chase their dreams because you only get one life and these realisations often don't come until it is too late. Only you are responsible for your mistakes and it is your duty to learn and better yourself from them.

To conclude, we all make mistakes, but it is rare that we learn from them before it is too late, I am fortunate that I have learned from mine. Every day is a school day for me now as I can see how oblivious I was before. As said by Moliere, 'it is not only for what we do that we are held responsible but also for what we do not do'. As the Irish saying goes, 'an rud is annamh is intact', the thing that is seldom is wonderful.

Task B: Essay Sample 11
Comment Set F

Society often teaches us that we ought to receive a particular set of experience for a specific age group that we are in. If we are toddlers, we gain our childhood experience by playing in the playgrounds and with other children. If we are teenagers, we are expected to have the experience of fulfilling our education and to achieve success. And, of course, when we are adults, we are deemed to be responsible enough to experience the world by travelling and meeting new people.

Unfortunately, I was not very lucky to have these set of experiences laid out in front of me. My parents passed away in a tragic plane crash when I was just ten years old. I was left to care for my two younger siblings who were aged three and four. I did not understand the dynamics of taking care of someone. I was often confused with numerous questions which were left unanswered. 'How do I care for them?', 'How do I put food on the table?', 'How am I supposed to know what a 3 and 4-years old need?'. These questions always left me frustrated and devastated. Many times, I felt that I should give up or the favourite question was 'Why me? Who decided that I would be the right person to bring my siblings up?'

Days would go by and I realised that my relatives were not very helpful as they could not assist my siblings and I financially. I started taking up odd jobs like to clean dishes or to repair watched to earn money to support my family. Financial aids would come from schools but it was never enough to buy the essentials, let alone my school books. Naturally, I dropped out of school at the age of 13. I worked full-time while my siblings studied. As if these days were not hard enough, my younger sister was diagnosed with a rare form of skin disorder, which caused her skin to peel off excessively, when she was just seven years old. I remember so vividly how I held her and cried as I felt extremely helpless.

It was then that I realised that stopping my education halfway was not going to help me in the long run. I may have money now but how was I going to support my family in the long run. I knew I had to be educated, I knew that I had to go to college so that I could secure myself a high-paying job in the future.

As my sister received treatments from community hospitals, I started studying part-time. I was sure not to neglect my family but at the same time achieve my dreams.

Today I am proud to say that if it was not for the tragic passing of my parents, I would have probably not known that I was this capable of being independent, supporting my family and caring for my sick sister. It was the childhood that I never had that taught me to be mature and responsible, to be loving yet strict. These experiences shaped me. They taught me not to find excuses and that I should make the most out of them. Most importantly, I can proudly say that it was my ill sister who was my inspiration to become a doctor. The experience of caring for her and also ensuring that I would be capable of caring for people who were just like her in the future shaped my determination and passion to get into medical school.

Now, life seems a little more settled as my sister has gotten better and my siblings have started working. As crazy as it may sound, when I look back, I would have not wanted life to be any other way. If it was, then I probably would have never become the compassionate, determined and knowledgeable person that I am today.

Comment Set G

Comment 1

The only way to get through life is to laugh your way through it.

****

Comment 2

I‘ve always thought that a big laugh is a really loud noise from the soul saying, “Ain‘t that the truth.”

****

Comment 3

Every survival kit should include a sense of humour.

****

Comment 4

There can never be enough said of the virtues, dangers, the power of a shared laugh.

Task B: Essay Sample 12
Comment Set G

Life is full of difficult times. There are stages, instances, moments in life where times are so difficult you are lost for words, lost for action, lost for thought. In these times, many believe that "The only way to get through life is to laugh your way through it".

I realised this on my first trip overseas alone. A spontaneous decision to travel to Cambodia with a volunteer company in an attempt to challenge myself. And a challenge it definitely was. My first day was an "introduction" day, and I was taken to the place where I would work 5 days a week for the next four weeks. The National Borey for Infants and Children was nothing like I had expected. There was limited information online, and all I knew was that the centre cared for one hundred and forty orphaned children living with disabilities. What I didn't know was that the kids shared a room with at least ten to twelve other kids, there was only one 'Mama' in each room who looked after all the kids, they all bathed each day in an outdoor area using buckets, they wore cloths as nappies, and so many more things that shocked me as I was taken on a tour around the centre. I left the centre feeling frightened, guilty, alone, sad, confused and all sorts of other emotions. I couldn't fathom the life these children had to live every single day.

I returned the day after for my first day of work in the physiotherapy room. Children were brought in, in groups, every hour between 8am and 4pm. But physiotherapy was prioritised for the children with severe physical disabilities only, most for those living with cerebral palsy. The children were brought in on wheelchairs that didn't fit them, and were placed anywhere on the floor where they could fit. The only instruction I got was to pick a child and start to stretch them. And that was what I did. For the first week, I was emotionally disconnected from the kids and I did what I was told. When walking home one day I noticed that there was music playing in the outdoor area and the kids that were able to stand and walk were dancing and playing. It was a sight that made me smile and feel warm inside, yet I felt saddened by the fact that this activity was only for the children who were able-bodied. After discussing with other volunteers, we went to the local markets and bought some cheap speakers that could connect to our phones. Of all the money I have ever spent, the seven dollars I spent on these fake speakers was the best decision I have ever made.

The first song we played was 'Gangnam style' by Psy and it was an absolute hit. A few of us held babies and danced with them, others sat behind older children and moved their arms with the music, and some danced with the children in their wheelchairs. The girl who we nicknamed 'Grumpy' smiled and laughed for the first time, the boy who sat in the corner and banged his head against the wall continuously stopped for at least sixty seconds and started laughing. The shared laughs around the room were contagious and I have never felt more accomplished. These kids, who were left stranded by their parents, who have lost so much in their lives already, who are unable to control their own limbs, were able to laugh through the pain and the sorrow. This became our goal from then on. Although I wanted help the children with their physical therapy, I knew that realistically, we didn't have the resources or the time to do so. In the short time that I had with them, laughter was the goal.

Francoise Sagan once said, "There can never be enough said of the virtues, dangers, the power of a shared laugh." I have never related to such a quote before. Just imagine if the world could refocus their time and energy into the happiness and laughter of those around them. If workplaces focused on the shared laughter rather than competition; productivity and efficiency of the team would skyrocket.

Task B: Essay Sample 13
Comment Set G

"The only way to get through life is to laugh your way through it"

Some say that time heals all wounds. This is true but it should be highlighted that laughter plays an important part in the healing process. Laughter is a critical component of the process of grieving the loss of a friend. I never really, truly, understood this sentiment until I experienced the loss of one of my closest friends.

Close to a year ago, my friend whom I had grown up with, got in his car, drove to a far-away beach and took his own life. He was 23 years young. I have experienced death before but it has never been sudden or self-inflicted. These experiences, although painful, were nothing on the scale of what my friends and I suffered and still do suffer.

Ironically, for a man who suffered from depression, he was probably one of the humorous persons I have known. He was one that could bring life to a party and bring humour to the even most dire (and often quite inappropriate) moments in our shared lives. The first time I travelled to the place where he passed was a pivotal point in truly understanding how important laughter is for grieving but also in the remembrance of my friend.

Seabird is a quiet coastal town, two hours north of Perth and boy was it a long two hours. Four of us made the trip North and for the latter half of the trip, it was silent. Upon arrival, we sat in silence for another hour contemplating what we had lost. Then almost like instinct, we began to reminisce about all these funny stories about my friend. Laughter broke out and it was almost like a weight had been lifted from our chests. On the way home we laughed and laughed, not only about those stories but other topics of interest.

Although I believe grieving is not a transient process, rather a lifelong experience, the use of laughter helps move the psyche from one of depression to one of acceptance and thus a critical component of the grieving process of losing a close friend.

Task B: Essay Sample 14
Comment Set G

The ability to laugh is a beautiful thing. It is a way that we as humans express our emotions of complete joy, our response to humour, and even our reaction to awkward and uncomfortable situations. There are many different meanings to a simple laugh, making it an extremely powerful and diverse emotion. I believe that having a sense of humour and sharing a laugh is invaluable, however, it can also be a dangerous way of human expression.

Laughing is one of the biggest means of sharing and expression the emotion of happiness, regardless of age or gender. In 2018, I was lucky to be participating in a clinical research trial at Liverpool hospital. My job involved interaction with patients, mainly recruiting them into the trial and thus explaining the medical procedure to them, including risks and obvious benefits. On one occasion I recruited a patient who was extremely ill, more than the other patients I had been involved with. As I ran through the motions, I introduced myself and began to explain the risks of the procedure and the purpose of the clinical trial that I was attempting to recruit him for. A huge grin emerged on his face and he began to chuckle to himself. He then said he felt so lucky to be talking to such a "young, healthy and talented young lady who has such a passion for what she does." I smiled back, thinking it was unusual for an elderly man in such a critical state to be smiling and laughing at a random girl he just met, right before his procedure that may or may not cure him.

There are certainly situations where laughing is the inappropriate expression to present, and I was in the mindset that this situation was one of them. I believe you must be emotionally aware of when it is suitable to share or express a laugh, as it may come across as insensitive or rude. Situations such as funerals, or important business meeting where you must be professional and act in a certain way for common courtesy and respect. This patient I was dealing with unfortunately passed away after the surgery as he could not be fixed. I came along with my supervising doctor to share the terrible news with the patient's family. At one point in the conversation, his family mentioned that they hoped he was "happy before entering the procedure", to which I replied that I had spoken to him for recruitment purposes and explained how he was smiling and laughing. The families' faces transformed from being broken and incredibly upset to short, small and respectful smile and laugh. They stated that he was an extremely happy man who always wanted to make light of situations and share happiness and positivity regardless of the situation.

It was at this moment that I finally understood the "power of a shared laugh." and smile. This patient was incredibly sick, yet he found it in him to smile and laugh in order to get through his situation and continue to spread happiness around him. This really stuck with me and allowed me to resonate with the fact that "every survival kit should include a sense of humour." I can now understand the reason he laughed and smiled during our conversation and realised it did make light of the situation. It had opened my eyes to the extreme positivity he was attempting to express.

Overall, sharing a laugh with your friends, family or even just an acquaintance is something we should all truly value as humans and understand the positivity it can express. Whilst there is indeed a time and a place for this, due to sensitive or formal situations where it can potentially have a negative impact, it is sometimes the only way to get through life. Laughing means you have a sense of humour and this is a very attractive and valuable trait to have. Moreover, we should all learn from this patient, share a laugh, make someone smile. You will not regret it!

Task B: Essay Sample 15
Comment Set G

The best medicine is laughter

"The only way to get through life is to laugh your way through it."

Creases formed on my father's forehead whilst he gently caressed my mother's cheeks with his emaciated fingers. He had definitely aged more than he should over the course of past few years. I observed him as he lifted her leg on his lap and softly kneaded her calves, all with a smile on his face. If you are unaware of the recent unfortunate event that transpired, you would definitely not be able to see through the smile he wore that day. I, on the other hand, could, the crow's feet that formed around his cheery eyes concealed the grief suppressed within.

Four years ago, my mother suffered a severe brain aneurysm, she was a foot from death's door. Doctors had delivered the distressing news that day and I remember being extremely concerned because I had never seen my father like that. I remember peeking through the slit of the bedroom door whilst he wept uncontrollably. He had intermittently let out a wail, abruptly gaining composure lest he alerted my sister and I.

I have always looked up to my parents and the love they have. Whilst they have had moments when all hell broke loose and blamestorming sessions followed, I witnessed the love they shared and showered each other. My father was the comedian and had always poked fun at my mother when the opportunity arose. My mother claimed that this really annoyed her but I could tell deep down she really loved his humour. He often cracked 'dad' jokes that my sister and I would patronisingly laugh at, nonetheless they always seem to lighten up any mood.

Three years into my mother's disability journey, I remember it was like any other day. We were having lunch and my father asked my mother if she would like to have some durian, my mother who has always been an avid durian lover, let out a yelp, "YES!". This was the first time my mother had spoken in three years. The brain bleed had been in the area of her speech and doctors had told us it was highly unlikely she would ever speak again. Whilst we were all in disbelief, we all cracked up in laughter at what had happened. I looked over at my father and for the first time in a long time he was laughing from within. In that moment, although temporary, my heart felt much lighter.

I will always remember the words my father brought me up with 'never take life too seriously, as you would never get out of it alive'. The more we embrace the humour, the more enjoyable our lives will become. The power of laughter is often discounted, if put to great use, could break boundaries and challenges we face. Thus, the best medicine for us all is indeed laughter.

Comment Set H

Comment 1

Where love rules, there is no will to power; and where power predominates, there love is lacking. The one is the shadow of the other.

****

Comment 2

Contrary to Pascal's saying, we don't love qualities, we love persons; sometimes by reason of their defects as well as of their qualities.

****

Comment 3

Love is like racing across the frozen tundra on a snowmobile which flips over, trapping you underneath. At night, the ice-weasels come.

****

Comment 4

They do not love that do not show their love. The course of true love never did run smooth. Love is a familiar. Love is a devil. There is no evil angel but Love.

Task B: Essay Sample 16
Comment Set H

Brotherly Love

Love, it may be argued, is the most powerful of human emotions. Love can make you swoon, act silly, love can make you run towards danger to protect a someone and it can make you give away your last dollar even though you need it. Love is a powerful emotion and it is one that during the course of their life almost every person will feel. Love comes in many shapes and sizes and can be viewed in many different contexts. Brotherly love in my view may be one of the strongest kinds of love there is.

The thing about a brother is that you don't get to pick them, either you arrive in this world and you have one from the moment you draw breath. Or one day you mum goes to the hospital and they arrive in this world and from then on you have one. If you are nearly the same age as your brother there's a good chance you do everything together. This is what happened to me.

When I was born, I already had a brother and at exactly the same time my brother got me. With only 18 months between us my brother and I were inseparable from the moment I could walk. We played together every day, we fought and wrestled, we watched cartoons and ate coco pops on weekends, he taught me how to ride my first bike. Then somewhere along the way we started to grow apart.

I think the moment it really started to happen was when we were in high school and I started to realise that the things we had previously had in common didn't really exist anymore. It wasn't sudden or dramatic it was more subtle and pernicious. We stopped spending as much time together, we talked less, confided in each other less and by the time I was 20 and he was 22 we barely spoke. In 2004 my brother moved from Australia to England and in 2005 shortly after I joined the military, he confided to my mother he was gay. To me this was not a shocking revelation, the shocking part for me was when my mother told me that one of the critical reasons he had waited until he had moved to England to tell people was because he was terrified of how I would react.

It took me a long time to reconcile in my mind that I had given him the impression that I would love him less because of his sexual preference. It devastated me that he had feared my reaction so much, for my part I didn't care what his sexual preference was, however, this was nearly impossible to explain to him. During 2005 following my first year in the military I returned home for Christmas, my brother was not there, however, I spoke to him on Christmas Day after he had spoken to Mum. Our conversation was long and in depth, I asked him why he had felt the way that he did, I explained my perspective and apologised for ever having given him the impression that I would love him less for who he was and we reconciled the damage that appeared to have been done to our relationship. During our conversation it became apparent to me that it would never matter what he did, who he was or who he chose to be with I would always love him. For me this realisation was a turning point in my understanding of what it is to love someone unconditionally. I fully understood the meaning of "Contrary to

Pascal's saying, we don't love qualities, we love persons; sometimes by reason of their defects as well as of their qualities".

Between my brother and I the experience of his quality of truth and my defect of perceived lack of acceptance we managed to find a strengthened bond through sharing and discussing how we felt. While it was unpleasant at time the experience that we had in 2005 was instrumental in bringing us back together after the emotional drift that we had experienced when we were in high school.

To me there may be no stronger love that the love experienced between two brothers. It is a love that means that you would do anything for them because you know they would do anything for you. One day when I am a father, I hope I have sons so that they too can experience the joy of what it is to have a brother, like I did.

Task B: Essay Sample 17
Comment Set H

Love

They say "Love is like racing across the frozen tundra on a snowmobile that flips over trapping you underneath. At night, the snow-weasels come." Ergo, love hurts, and I learnt this the hard way.

There is a great discrepancy between love and infatuation. Infatuation connotes loving qualities of a person, idealising them, putting them on a pedestal and being blind to their flaws; the epitome of "la vie en rose." However, love is much more profound; it is to see someone in their entirety, flaws and all, and love them. It is unconditional positive regard and genuine empathy; to truly love is to make reciprocal compromises and sacrifices for their sake. Love brings out the best of in both people.

My first relationship was fiery, passionate and a short-lived archetype of blind infatuation. I met him in my first year of Uni. In the beginning it was full of bliss; I remember those lazy summer days lounging under the forget-me-not blue sky, those romantic walks in the city at night, those adoring conversations until 4am… He gave me the attention I craved, made me feel desired and gave me a taste of wild adventure. I was blissfully in love and relishing the prospect that there was someone out there who reciprocated my feelings.

Eventually, my infatuation compelled me to restructure all elements of my life around him. My sole purpose of going to university was to spend time with him and I suddenly found no more time for anything else. I kept denying this nagging sense of emptiness within me, that little voice which whispered that I was doing nothing novel in my life, nothing to challenge myself or to stimulate self-growth. Eventually, I became so emotionally invested in this one pillar of my life that all the other people in my life receded from me.

Thus, when this one supporting pillar gave way, my whole world crumbled. He had to move interstate for a new degree, but gave up on the relationship because he did not want to commit to a long-distance relationship. Shards of ice pierced my heart and gnawed at it. The culmination of my emotional investment in him, then ultimately being rejected by the one person I relied on was a devastating blow to my ego to say the least. I cycled through a medley of emotions: despair, to wistfulness of what may have been, anger at myself for not keeping a firmer hold on him, and eventually I plunged into loneliness.

It was through travelling and time that I drew on the privilege of hindsight to plant the seeds of my recovery. Initially the void in my life was unbearable; my thoughts kept flying back to him but my mind refrained because it was too painful. But I eventually realised that the entire relationship was comprised of my delusions due to infatuation. I had overlooked numerous flaws, such as his proclivity to rage which rendered us incompatible. Instead of voicing my feelings, I suppressed them to avoid conflict. I recall that I accepted all his decisions without question or opinion, to which he appreciated me for my submissive nature as it only reasserted his dominance. In an attempt to appease his temperamental, uncompromising and egocentric nature, I had unknowingly relinquished my autonomy and spirit; and I just because I craved the feeling of being "cherished" by someone else. I had been infatuated with him, and it cost me my identity.

For so long, my self-worth was contingent upon his validation so the first person I had to reconcile with was myself. I took steps towards self-growth by engaging in activities I suddenly found I had time for. I immersed myself in Russian literature, hiked with friends to secluded places, learnt how to bake a mean chicken pie, participated in a research course and even volunteered to advocate oral health at the Homeless Connect. I picked up the pieces of my life by travelling to Vietnam, reconnecting with my extended family and just by wandering around ancient towns and learning about my culture. I felt my self-confidence grow with every step and I was slowly able to rediscover my sense of self and my love for life.

Love is meant to help and not hurt. By realising this, I was emancipated from its chains. By acknowledging my blind infatuation, excessive tolerance and loss of autonomy in that relationship, I experienced self-growth and eventually took steps to rediscovering my sense of self. I learnt that my personal happiness is not contingent on another person; the first person you need to be in love with is yourself. For now, I will take some time out to learn some more skills, and enjoy life without the dependence of another. In the future, when I am ready, I certainly hope that I will choose someone who has more respect for me.

Task B: Essay Sample 18
Comment Set H

Modern society is notorious for their superficial and romantic definition of 'love'. They often see it as being the spark between two people. However, love should be seen in the light that Romantic poets such as William Wordsworth wrote about. Love should be properly defined as a union between people and Nature. As Carl Jung very elegantly and beautifully expressed it, "Where love rules, there is no will to power; and where power predominates, there love is lacking. The one is the shadow of the other." This quote superbly demonstrates the union that love entails. When true love exists within anyone, they are at one with the people and Nature, and our intrinsic thirst for power and control disappears.

True love is quite rare in our modern world. Even the most powerful leaders such as the president of the United States of America and the Prime Minister of the United Kingdom fail time and time again to demonstrate their love for their people. It is scary because, without proper love from our leaders, they are disconnected from us and they thirst for control and power often by being secretive or by twisting truths. A leader who truly loved their people shouldn't feel powerful or the need to control, but instead, an overwhelming urge to guide and to serve.

Personally, I experienced the change of superficial love to true love through my father. I remember when I was young that he would often express his 'love' to me through buying me presents or giving me hugs. However, he would continually use his power of being 'dad' time and time again to make me do things or make me change. There was indeed a disconnection, a lack of a union between my father and myself. On the surface, to any of friends or more remote family, it would seem that our relationship was that of an idealistic father-son union. However, there was always a lack of respect and appreciation between us. As we both grew older and matured, he began to realise that materialistic happiness wasn't enough for his son and that our relationship was thinning and our communication was becoming more limited as the months went on. We both needed to redefine the love we superficially expressed towards each other. My father relinquished his position of power as 'dad' which all parents should do and came to a level of mutual respect with me. Instead of the demands, there would be discussion and instead of controlling the direction of my future he would gently advise but always ended it by saying, "I'll support your choices, whatever they may be." My experience of this proper love allowed me to open up and finally reconnect with my father.

Although my experience of love was personal, it doesn't change the fact that this proper love which my father now expressed to me created a union where we were all on the same level. His power to control and dominate was gone and my power to threaten to leave or never talk to him again disappeared. Although love and hate are often described as polar opposites, love and power can also be seen as two ends of a spectrum. Every bit of power we are willing to relinquish towards a person, individuals, a group or even nature we instantly become more loving in the true Romantic sense as described by numerous of Wordsworth's poems. This unique connection to someone or something is an act of surrender. Modern society must come to realise that love and power cannot go together. We must redefine 'love' by relinquishing our thirst for power and control, for only then we can truly love and be loved.

Comment Set I

Comment 1

There are people who have money and there are people who are rich.

****

Comment 2

After a certain point, money is meaningless. It ceases to be the goal. The game is what counts.

****

Comment 3

It's a kind of spiritual snobbery that makes people think they can be happy without money.

****

Comment 4

While money can't buy happiness, it certainly lets you choose your own form of misery.

Task B: Essay Sample 19
Comment Set I

Money can buy happiness.

Working on the ambulances in the busy streets of London taught me a lot. Mostly it taught me how disconnected I was. Reflecting on it, it reminds me how disconnected I still am. I was, and am, in many ways a snob. Most of us are.

The seed of this realisation was planted, nurtured, ruptured and flourished in the space of two hours. That's the glory of ambulance work.

I was sitting on a park bench with a homeless man called Joe. A good Samaritan had passed Joe by whilst he was asleep on the bench and decided in all of their good will that he was dead, so they called an ambulance. Unfortunately, their good will did not extend to actually nudging Joe, which would have awoken him from his slumber and highlighted the key piece of information that Joe was in fact not dead. Instead, they walked on by, undoubtedly with a proud smirk spreading across their cheeks.

So here I was, having woken Joe, sitting next to him while he smoked a cigarette and I filled out some paperwork. I'd met Joe on the job a few times and he was a hard man. In his words, our educations differed primarily in that I went to university and he went to the school of “hard-knocks”. Scars and stone-cold eyes were proof enough.

Joe was admiring my new haircut and shiny boots when he chuckled and said, “Man, you’ve got it made.”

“How do you figure?” I asked.

“Clean head, clean boots, clean clothes, you’ve reached the end of the rainbow.” Joe replied.

I was perplexed. By no means did any of these things resonate for me as worthy of comparison to gold, especially not the mythical kind found at the end of the rainbow. These were material things that in my spiritual superiority I had labelled as insignificant, trivial.

I laughed and remarked that these things didn’t really matter.

Joe’s convivial mood quickly turned sullen. He scoffed, shook his head and took a deep inhale of his cigarette.

“If those things don’t matter, let’s swap. Boots for boots. Clean shave for dread-locks. C’mon...” Joe was fixating in his gaze. His look revealed no sign of a joke.

I laughed uncomfortably, replying that “You know these are my work boots, I can’t just give them up.”

“Would you though? I mean if you were allowed to, would you?” Joe asked, still staring directly at me.

I looked at his boots. They were moist and one didn’t even have a sole. I suddenly became aware of the distinct smell of urine radiating of his jacket, and possibly even his hair. I’d been told by a homeless patient a couple of weeks back that on weekends people would walk down alleyways while intoxicated and urinate on the rough sleepers. Whether this smell was from Joe or a stranger, I couldn’t say, and probably neither could he.

“No, Joe, I wouldn’t.” I sighed.

I always chanted that money can’t buy happiness and the value of material things comes only out of capitalist conditioning and the desire to fill the bottomless pits of human suffering. It sounded pretty out-there and always went down a treat at the pub, but was that what I actually believed? And besides, who was I to talk about the importance of money? I had grown up in an upper-middle class family and went to a private school in a nice neighbourhood just outside of Melbourne. I had never had a need for money. There had never been any threat of hunger, thirst or homelessness. I realised then that I was privileged because I had never needed to think about these things. I've always, as Joe says, had it made.

With more money Joe would be warm, fed, healthy and clean. He would be able to find work and develop a meaningful life. I have not made an assumption about the meaning of Joe's life, it was he who told me on a previous encounter that his life had no meaning. This was while I bandaged his arms after a failed suicide attempt.

The belief that money doesn't buy happiness is, as the saying goes, "spiritual snobbery", and it is held only by those who have never experienced a life without it.

I often think about Joe and where life has taken him, and when I do every cell in my body hopes that he has more money, because I like Joe, and I want him to have a better life.

Task B: Essay Sample 20
Comment Set I

The Divorce

It was drizzling outside and as I meticulously observed each droplet, I could visualise my life unfolding in the background. A corporate 9-5 job may be satisfying at the financial front but was I truly content with my life? I wanted to believe that the money I earned made me 'rich' but did it? Was my life indulged in beautiful moments and memories that would construct my future or was I slaving away for paper notes? The problem was not with my job for I enjoyed it but the fact that I didn't a life apart from it and perhaps that's why my wife divorced me.

The grey, wispy clouds mirrored my thoughts that snow-balled into fears. A moment whisked me away. I imagined Henry growing up to be a young boy giving his speech at his graduation. Would I really be a part of this achievement? I had already neglected him, disappeared from his childhood where I should have been helping him tie his shoelaces, riding a bike or kicking a ball. Instead, memories of the nanny and my wife, erupted. I can imagine the bitter pang and shame of not having a father at Sports Day to cheer one on. It breaks me to think that in my son's most impressionable age I was not there for him. My job had always taken a priority and perhaps my wife's decision to take a divorce was not unwarranted. I hate to think that my son may have felt unloved watching one parent do their duty, I hate to think what he may have thought about me in those precious moments?

It was getting darker outside and my computer screen blacked out. My thoughts, evaporated deeper into my fears. My wife and the love and attention I had failed to provide her. Perhaps that had led her to cheat on me? I wanted to blame myself, but I could not fathom her with another man. It disgusted me. I understand her anger and pain, yet she could have come to me about it before committing such an act of betrayal. Regardless, I will regret moments spent without her. I will regret not eating with her at the breakfast table because I ate at work. Work, work, work is what my passion was, what I had always immersed myself in, to the point where I had forgotten I had a family. I will regret being too busy for date nights. Time, is all she wanted. More time. A request so simple yet so profound. All I could think about was rising in my ranks at work. I wanted to do well for myself and for my family. But this thought had ended up corrupting our entire life.

The day my wife had divorced me, I felt as if someone had pulled a rug from under my chair. My life had collapsed and more so when I found out about her betrayal. Although, that did mitigate my guilt. Perhaps, my wife never really loved me and the 'time' concept was her idea of concealing the truth. Nevertheless, I had a duty towards my son. I was still a father and wanted to be a prominent part of his life. I wanted to start fresh. For my son to forgive and forget. But I was not sure how I should go about contacting him. 'Henry, I'm terribly sorry,' 'Are you OK,' or 'Hey, how are you?' I wish the pain could disappear in a crevice in the ground forever, out of sight and out of mind. In the end I texted him, 'Hey, miss you son.' And the reply, 'I miss you too,' was enough to restore hope in me. I may have been clutching at straws but I knew in the end I would float.

Task B: Essay Sample 21
Comment Set I

The Expense of Misery

I walk down the streets of the city's outskirts, in a suburb gracefully plagued with multi-million dollars estates. At this time of the afternoon, one would expect the BMWs to rush down from work, one would hear the symphonies of piano and clarinet pieces buzz around - played by children from those rich households. One would expect a vibrant, rich atmosphere, reflective of the neatly trimmed front yards and golden fences lining the sides of the street.

But today was different, almost dismal.

The news from a few days ago has spread to the media. People from this suburb and nearby has learnt of the "unimaginable", an event so unexpected to happen in this affluent area. As I stroll down the streets towards my house, I reflect on such a shocking event that has impacted me. I can only think that money indeed, cannot buy happiness, but it only lets one choose their own form of misery.

During my first year in primary school, there was a fairly quiet but very generous kid who we all called Frankie. Every lunchtime, he would have 10 packets of chocolate truffles, and handed them out to the school of friends that followed him. He would boast about his gaming collection in class, describing newly released, expensive video games and gadgets other kids only could dream of. Frank would always rush to the canteen, buying more food than he could fit, only giving them away to fellow students inevitably.

I would sometimes join in and be the opportunist too, scabbing a fair share of his goods and imagining the amazing quality of living in a rich household.

Never did I know, I was entirely wrong.

It was not until the 5th year of primary when I realised Frank only lived a few blocks from me. Although just a few blocks apart, we were from very different households, in fact, a very different suburb. His affluent suburb made a discriminating socioeconomic border with mine, but nevertheless, we became close with more frequent meet ups. He would invite me to his house at occasions, where I witnessed the deluxe array of marble furniture, played his exquisite arsenal of games and slowly became a lowly member of his elegant mansion.

However, as we eventually grew up, past high school, there was something about him that changed.

No longer was he a reserved individual. Instead, he would constantly rant about how his parents have been favouring his older brother, giving him financial support that he never has access to. He would complain with fire and maliciousness about how his parents were the true faces of evil and injustice, how they would neglect him as an unwanted scion.

"No more games! You have grown up! I am not spending anything else for you!" he would imitate with utmost hatred.

Yells of abuse and cries of panic became a regular resident of his household as I passed by his house.

His rage spread like wildfire and I constantly reminded him if everything was okay, only to no avail.

He would have stages of mania, where his temperament ran insane like a wild predator.

Then the inevitable happened - gunshots were heard a few nights ago, reportedly in the Noble household. It was later revealed that Frank murdered his father before releasing the trigger next to his temple.

I stroll down the streets, regretting not taking action before. Everything, however, happened very unexpectedly and shockingly, even I could not have imagined. I kept strolling, thinking about how money is indeed such a harmful substance, how it forms the fundamental pit of misery and heinousness. I have always considered my living conditions as horrendous when compared with Frank's, but now my views have changed completely.

Comment Set J

Comment 1

There are things known and there are things unknown, and in between are the doors of perception.

****

Comment 2

After all, life is really simple; we ourselves create the circumstances that complicate it.

****

Comment 3

The difference between who you are and what you want to be is what you believe you can do.

****

Comment 4

Overthinking is the art of creating problems that weren't even there.

Task B: Essay Sample 22
Comment Set J

We humans are fascinating creatures, we are privileged to be able to speak, see, hear, touch and smell but, somehow our ability to distort our perceptions deceive us. We are masters of overthinking and ruining our great moments on this earth. We are born to run and play and absorb the beauties that mother nature has bestowed upon us but, for some reason the devil inside us doesn't want us to experience those gems.

When I was 2, my parents left me with grandparents in India and moved to New Zealand. 15 years passed by, I had not seen my parents since the day the boarded the plane, I had become accustomed and content with my current way of life. My grandparents were my everything. They fed me, walked me to school and took me to Bharatanatyam lessons (classical Indian dance). We lived in a low to middle class neighbourhood where everyone knew everyone's names. Every Saturday afternoon, the children that lived on my street would come over to my house and we would watch a Malayalam movie. That is because we were the only household that owned a television set. I loved living like this, I was living in a neighbourhood and in a household where I was wanted. I couldn't imagine a better life than that (only because I was oblivious to the standards of living beyond the walls of my little community).

One eerie night, we received a phone call on the landline which had started piling with dust since, we never received phone calls. We were all taken aback by the ringing, my grandmother slowly picked up the phone and that is when my life changed forever. Her daughter in law, my mother, was on the other end of the call. She hadn't spoken to her in 13 years but, she was calling to let us know that my dad was in a serious car crash and that he was in a coma. I was never curious about my parents. I didn't even know where they lived. I wasn't interested in knowing the people that abandoned me. However, that night my chest felt very heavy, I was filled with sorrow but I never knew how that was even possible. My grandma told me to just ignore it and carry on with my life. I assumed it was because she was mad at her son for abandoning his only child and leaving the country to live a better life. As the night grew darker, I was racking my brain wondering why they had called and whether my grandma was withholding any more information about what happened on the phone call. 'Maybe they wanted to see me', 'maybe my mum was moving back to India'. I spent the whole night overthinking the situation.

When morning came, I told my grandma that I wanted to go to New Zealand to meet them. She refused at first but after throwing a fit, she finally decided to let me go. Both my grandparents weren't healthy enough to come with me so, they decided to let me go on my own.

My grandma wrote down the name of the hospital and told me to take a taxi once I got there. After a 20-hour plane ride and an 1 hour taxi ride, I finally reached the hospital but it turned out that my dad had passed away the night before and my mum had left without any trace. I was so lost and disappointed. She knew I was coming but, didn't wait around to see me. Once again, I felt abandoned and this time I can't blame anyone else but myself. They never asked to see me but I did it anyway and I got my heart broken.

I used to be a little girl, leading a peaceful life but, now I am troubled by mistakes that I created.

Comment Set K

Comment 1

Any old place [he] can hang [his] hat is home sweet home.

****

Comment 2

It takes hands to build a house, but only heart can build a home.

****

Comment 3

Home is the starting place of love, hope and dreams.

****

Comment 4

There's no place like home.

Task B: Essay Sample 23
Comment Set K

Of Bikes and Cakes

Today, my boyfriend broke up with me. I wanted so much to run home and tell my mum and dad how much I was in pain, but I couldn't. They are miles away from where I am now. So I took out my bike and pedalled mu blues away around the block.

I remember how my now ex-boyfriend actually found it ridiculous that I'd still hang my childhood bide in the apartment. Now I understand how the presence of that bike around makes me feel like I never really left home. It constantly reminds me of the first time my dad taught me how to ride the bike, how he was patient and reassuring; and how he promised he would never let me down. Today, that sense of security – of making me feel that despite the heartbreak, life will eventually get better – came handy. To my dad's eyes, I will always be the best girl and he will always have my back.

When I returned to the apartment, I decided, "I should bake a cake!" And while mixing the flour and sugar and eggs, all my childhood memories with mum came rushing in…

In grade school, I used to wear thick glasses and braces, and kids at school would tease me with all sorts of hurtful names like nerdy, ugly daisy, just to name a few. I felt like an outcast. But every time I got home, mum, upon hearing my footsteps at the door, would exclaim, "My beautiful princess is home! Now let's bake this princess a cake." All the pain I felt during those days would instantly disappear. At home, I was royalty – with the tastiest cake in the world on the platter! – regardless of my appearance.

So I had my slice of cake today. I can't say it stopped m from crying over my boyfriend's rejection. But then again, it made me felt right at home in the warmth of my mother's arms. I knew the 'princess' in me will never be beaten emotionally – at least, not for long.

It is this acceptance that William Jerome speaks of when he mentioned that "Any old place [he] can hang [his] hat is home sweet home". Just like the house I currently live in is not my childhood home, it is the memories I bring in it that makes me feel like I never really left home.

Home is where I can retreat at the end of the day: a secure heaven, filled with love and free from judgement. It is my own space, a space I choose to share with those I love, and those who love me in return. It is the love and simplicity of my childhood memories that make a home: a haven of memories, my mother tenderly teaching me to bake a cake, or dad teaching me to ride a bike; promising he would never let go.

Task B: Essay Sample 24
Comment Set K

Throughout life and its many experiences, many of us move houses, cities, states or countries; but coming back to any previous home always fills us with some little bit of warmth. The truth, time and time again, is that home is found because of the people and the memories; not the materials or the locations. With the right company, we can find a home on Mars or the moon if we wanted to.

The idea that "it takes hands to build a house, but only hearts can build a home" reminds me of the book Samurai's Garden. In this novel, the main character Stephan is forced to leave his home in New York and go to Japan for the summer. At first, he is extremely upset and unwilling to open up his mind to the experience that is ahead of him. Throughout the novel, he meets several people and forms several deep, meaningful friendships. By the end of the novel, through a beautiful telling of the story of Stephan's life in which readers personally connect to the characters, the author makes the point to the reader that home is truly where such relationships are made and experiences are felt. This is done through exploring Stephan's hesitation and internal conflict of returning back to New York, the place he considered home, as he will be leaving his newfound family behind.

Home need not be through real-life relationships but can be felt through connections to television shows or movies as well. Another example of how homes are created by people and experience is the television show Gilmore Girls. The show is set in a small town and follows the lives of a mother and her daughter. Throughout the show, viewers are also exposed to all of the characters within the town, each with their own quirks and characteristics. Add in the music and the fast-paced sarcastic dialogue and every viewer becomes hooked. No matter how long it has been since I have seen an episode, I start to feel the nostalgia of returning home and meeting the characters, when I watch one.

Thus it is evident that home is not determined by location, space, or other physical attributes. Home is where one makes friends, lives life experiences, grows into a better person, makes memories, and so much more. It has everything to do with one's heart and the hearts of those around them, and this is what makes the feeling of home one of the most special feelings of all time.

Task B: Essay Sample 25
Comment Set K

Home is essential in our lives; it is where we can be our own selves and free to do the things we want to do. Having a home gives us a feeling of comfort and security. However, like many material possessions, a physical home is something that we may not be able to keep forever. Such was my experience when we migrated to Australia and left our home overseas.

I struggled to overcome the feeling of "homesickness" and it took me quite a while to feel at home in a new country. My first few weeks in Australia were hard for me. From a two-storey, five-bedroom house overseas, we moved to a three-bedroom apartment in Sydney. I used to have my own room. This time, I had to share my bedroom with my younger sister. I used to ask mum why we had to sacrifice our big house for a small apartment in Sydney. She kept on reminding me that physical things in life can fade or be taken away from me, hence, I should focus on the intangible ones and be not attached to our old home overseas.

I started reflected on our old home. Why was it so valuable to me? How could I develop the same feeling to our new home? Then I realised that it was not the aesthetics and the space or measurements of the house. I liked our old house and valued it because that was where I grew up and all my childhood memories were there. Having said that, I shook my head and recognised that memories stay in the heart and soul, not in a physical house. It is something that I could bring with me all the time.

I began helping out mum in "building" our new home. Aside from buying appliances and furniture, I also added the care, love, and family spirit in our new home. I realised that what I needed was just right next to me: my family to complete the corners of our home; and the healthy family bonding and long-lasting memories we share together, which light up our home. Since then, I felt complete, I felt at home and there was no longer a feeling of homesickness.

As a multicultural country, Australia has a huge number of migrants from around the world, and many are yet to arrive here. They might face the same struggle as I had when I first moved here. In order to overcome this, they may do the same thing as I did; that is, to build the home in their hearts and souls. Through this, I was able to have an irrevocable condition of having a home to myself. I can go from one place to another, bringing my own home with me, as I have made a home for myself inside my heart and souls and found the things needed to furnish it.

Comment Set L

Comment 1

'Age is an issue of mind over matter, if you don't mind, it doesn't matter'

Mark Twain

Task B: Essay Sample 26
Comment Set L

I know it's Cliché…

Sometimes I forget what Mark Twain taught me - 'age is an issue of mind over matter, if you don't mind, it doesn't matter'. Daily reminders of this would be ideal as a young adult. The famous saying that age is just a number means a lot in the years of development. I am a big believer that the number of candles on the cake each year should not determine your lifestyle, what stage of life you are at or hobbies you have, etc. Whether you are eighteen going to college or fifty, what does it matter? Both students will come out with the same diploma, subject to passing exams, but not subject to what birthday you last celebrated. Everyone will have a unique journey through life, and that is absolutely okay and makes life that bit more interesting.

I am at the stage of life where I am continuously finding myself in environments where I am the youngest, according to my age. A prime example being work. As a result, I can relate on quite a personal level to being looked down on by others due to my age. Some people, who I have grown to learn are simply ill-educated, believe you are your age and just because they're older than you, they somehow have the right to talk down to you and in a disrespectful manner. I have had scenarios where patients request to speak to another member of administrative staff. I can see in their eyes and their tone of voice that it is because of my young appearance giving away that I am younger than my colleagues. For some reason, these people believe just because I haven't been on earth for as long as the others, I can't do my job to the same ability, despite having received the same training. It can be quite distracting and discouraging when this happens but it has forced me to be a little more thick skinned. In an attempt to find a silver lining to such unpleasant encounters, I am glad that I am able to recognise such situations and know that it is wrong to treat someone else with such disrespect. Having experienced the upsetting but enraging feeling of being belittled, I wouldn't wish it on my worst enemy. I can only hope that when I am older, I can remember this feeling and refrain from acting in such a manner.

Although different stages of life are present, they should not be dictated by a number. I do wish that later in my life, I am able to look back and reflect on my life. To say I have achieved all the things I once dreamed of would be the ultimate goal, like getting married, becoming a parent and getting my dream job. I do believe where you end up later in life is a reflection of your journey and the experiences you were subjected to in youth. I mean if this wasn't true, what would be the point of all the studying and hard grind. The majority of my life, so far, has been based on studying and saving money to be able to go to college so that I can get a good job to be able to live a good life and provide for my family down the line. I sure hope that the sacrifices made in youth pay off in due course. What still stands is that there is no age dictations on which order you must live your life in or how another individual should treat you at each stage of life. Coincidently, how we treat others is a reflection of the youth we live through.

We often hear that we must not let a diagnosis define us. In a similar way, we must not let a number define us. If one wants to return to education later in life, or retire early or get a tattoo at the age of 80, fair play! As long as we treat others with respect and are happy, I don't see any problem. There is no handbook to living. I think a lot of people could benefit from a gentle reminder that, it is okay to do life "backwards".

Comment Set M

Comment 1

Fantasy is a way of understanding reality.

****

Comment 2

Fantasy is no more than escapism.

****

Comment 3

Imagination is one of the most important kinds of thinking.

****

Comment 4

Sympathy and empathy are dependent on imagination.

Task B: Essay Sample 27
Comment Set M

The ability to Dream the impossible, see the unseeable and feel things you are yet to experience is surely one of the greatest gifts that could be bestowed upon someone. I believe my personal happiness and success in life and career can be in part attributed to my ability to imagine form and feel deeply.

From the age I finally made that leap into fluency as a reader I spent many hours lost in books. Hours in buses, trains or waiting for life to happen where spent in happiness inhaling the words of the author rather than in board frustration. Many of the great interests of my life as well as beliefs are centered in the page of books I read as a child and young adult. Wilbur Smith , I have a great to deal to thank you for! Images of Elephants and stories of ancient people and beautiful landscapes pepper my mind. My imagination running freely gave me happiness at the time as well as forging a great interest in the continent. In 2012 my feet landed on Kenyan soil after some 35 years of dreaming of this most incredible place. My time in Africa is now a treasured memory that lives alongside my memories of the books that created the imagination and drive to go there in the first place.

As a first year physiotherapy student I was asked what I thought where the qualities that would make a good therapist. What is it that you could strive for that could make you better? Along with all the obvious choices regarding clinical reasoning etc. I stated that I believed understanding your patient was important. 20 years later I still believe this to be true in fact I believe it is critical to being good at what I do.

Empathy, the ability to feel what your patient feels and to share their journey is both the joy and occasionally heartbreak of my career. Empathy goes beyond just having an appreciation for someone's physical pain. Knowing what a dislocated shoulder or any number of examples I can physically directly relate to is very useful but not the empathy that requires imagination . This Empathy is the ability to listen to your patients' personal stories and actually imagine what it's like to be in their world and feel what they feel. This is skill that can't be taught and is fully dependent on imagination. I could write a thesis on the stories I have heard over the last 20 years of my career. Talking and listening to my patients is the true joy of my day to day. Being swept into the adventure of my 72 years married couples' immigration to Australia on a boat with 6 months old twins evokes joy and happiness in my heart. The memory of listening to my patient explain how she sits in her car with her mask on for 10 minutes to allow the fear and memory of her violent assault and rape to pass before stepping out into the world still has the power to move me to tears.

In conclusion I am eternally grateful for my imagination and the skill of empathy it awards me. Without the ability to create those pictures and feelings in my head the world would have been a very dull place for me.

Comment Set N

Comment 1

Music is never meant for us to control it, but to be swept away by it.

****

Comment 2

There are monsters and there are demons and music can keep one at bay while invoke the other.

****

Comment 3

Music is the universal language of mankind.

****

Comment 4

The purpose of music is to release us from the tyranny of conscious thoughts.

Task B: Essay Sample 28
Comment Set N

Music – the breath to life

There are many aspects that connect us together in life, but is there one tool that holds a universal language and binds us together? Music – it is the vessel that takes us to places of escape and connects humankind. To begin, although styles of music have greatly evolved throughout the centuries, the core of its power remains the same – to entertain and provide individuals with a safe space to escape a difficult reality. Additionally, as a ubiquitous language, music delivers the blanket of comfort to unite humanity and remind us of the goodness in life.

Firstly, music is a medium that that can help us escape the difficulties of daily life and help us to reconnect with our true selves. Different beliefs and how individuals react to the world around them reflects diversity in humanity. Despite these differences guiding presuppositions about each other and how we perceive ourselves, however, music can mould who we are and help us escape reality. In particular, when we listen to music that triggers feelings of happiness and joy, our fears, insecurities and worries are momentarily washed away. When iconic music groups, such as 5 Seconds of Summer and BTS produce and perform their music, they are trailblazers in the music industry. Through their artistic work, they create an identity of community-like connections amongst themselves and their diverse audience. Their sense of originality in lyrics that speak of self-love and self-acceptance is extended through their charitable work in Friends with Friends and Love Yourself campaigns to help the youth find comfort through difficult times. Such music that reflects everyday struggles and the musicians who devote their craft into connecting with their fans through true to life lyricism and production gives individuals the temporary relief from the reality of hardships. Hence, music is not only a form of entertainment, but also provides a safe space to deeply reconnect with ourselves.

Furthermore, the universal language of music brings comfort in times of need to remind us of the resilience of humanity. Socialising maintains bonds between individuals, strengthening one's affiliation with others. Similarly, music is one of many languages that helps connect humanity together and bring a sense of belonging. Such an impact reflects the high social value that music can bring comfort through unity. This is evidenced through the Fire Fight Australia concert in 2020 and the Red Cross Flood Appeal concert in 2022. These events highlight the ubiquitous nature of music that brings strength to communities and reflects the enduring nature of the resilient human spirit to overcome the tragedies of natural disasters of bushfires and floods. Additionally, the Global Citizens Organisation runs a global campaign to end extreme poverty, by hosting global concerts that feature well-known artists. Such communal gatherings have positive intentions of raising funds and awareness, calling individuals to act on their roles as global citizens and pay it forward. Such unity 4 comes from the universal language of music, which is the instigator behind achieving collective change to put forth actions of good intentions and make affirmative changes in society. Thus, music provides humanity with a language of collective resilience and togetherness through trials that test our capabilities.

In conclusion, music provides us with a route of escape and greater our connection with each other. Firstly, lyrics and music production have the power to momentarily relieve us from difficulties and hardships of day to day reality. Additionally, music is the universal language that binds us together, bringing comfort and building resilience to overcome tragedies. Music truly gives meaning to life.

Comment Set O

Comment 1

Music is the universal language of mankind.

****

Comment 2

There are monsters and there are demons, and music can keep one at bay while invoke the other.

Comment 3

The purpose of music is to release us from the tyranny of conscious thought.

****

Comment 4

Behind one's favourite song is an untold story.

Task B: Essay Sample 29
Comment Set O

The Music Through our Veins

Music has been enjoyed by many for a long time. From the public houses of Olde England to the modern times of one's own motor vehicle, many have enjoyed the tunes and melodies of music. However, music can have deeper purposes and effects. It can calm tense situations and bridge previously insurmountable emotional chasms between peoples. As such, although music may be for pure enjoyment, it can also serve more sublime purposes.

Music can be just for pure enjoyment. In Medieval times, music was enjoyed from courtly palaces to public houses and in the streets and homes of ordinary people. Nowadays too, music is enjoyed in people's houses and in public venues. Not many think too deeply about it. It can be used for dancing, for singing, or just to be listened to for enjoyment and relaxation. And what is wrong with that?

However, music can also serve deeper, more sublime purposes. For example, it can calm violent spirits and also be a universal language that bridges previously insurmountable gaps between peoples. For example, one may read the storey of David and King Saul, in the Old Testament, and how the latter was in a foul and violent mood. Sensing this, David played on his harp and calmed the spirits of Saul, thus averting a potential disastrous situation. Indeed, such logic has been used nowadays in public places where delinquents tend to congregate, such as train stations and outside shopping centres. Outside such places, the owners have tried playing classical music and, as a result, they have found the incidence of crimes at these venues has decreased. Secondly, music can be used as a universal language. For example, about 3 years ago, a music ensemble form the US visited North Korea. They played many pieces, including the North Korean national anthem to a crowd of North Korean leaders. The latter were seen on TV emotionally moved, some even crying from this. Indeed, it can be seen how music can also serve as a universal language that is able to bridge emotional gaps between seemingly diametrically opposite peoples, if but for a moment in time. As such, music can serve important and transcending purposes.

In conclusion, although music can serve as simple enjoyment, it can also serve more sublime purposes, such as soothing violent spirits and bridging gaps between peoples. Music has been a form of pure and simple enjoyment for generations of human-kind. However, music has also served deeper purposes. It has been used to help calm people and prevented potentially violent situations. It has also served as a universal language that has helped to bridge gaps between different peoples.

Comment Set P

Comment 1

Forgiveness is a virtue of the brave.

Indira Gandhi

****

Comment 2

It is easier to forgive an enemy than to forgive a friend.

William Blake

****

Comment 3

You can make up a quarrel, but it will always show where it was patched.

Edgar Watson Howe

****

Comment 4

To err is human; to forgive, divine.

Alexander Pope

****

Comment 5

There is no revenge so complete as forgiveness.

Josh Billings

Task B: Essay Sample 30
Comment Set P

My interpretation of forgiveness is to accept any injustice and wrongdoing that has been inflicted upon you that would have caused you pain and hurt. Acknowledge the negative feelings and appreciate that responding in kind with acts of revenge will only encourage the continuation of further negative energy being permeated out into the world. God knows we have enough anger, and revenge being carried out in the world right now. You only have to look at the endless stream of negative comments furnishing social media responses and new phrases being invented, such as revenge porn. My philosophy and general rule are to follow the adage of "taking the moral high ground".

Extending the theme of revenge to nations, the conflict between Israel and Palestine exemplifies the never-ending acts of revenge that have only caused misery and death.

At the level of the individual, forgiving someone however does not mean that you must maintain a relationship with that person and keep them within your social circle. You must protect yourself from further hurt and pain. Forgiving someone and forgetting is not brave but an act of stupidity. Forgetting about past injustices that you suffer from only makes you vulnerable to future injustices and disrespect being committed against you. The adage also that I live by is "Fool me once, shame on you, fool me twice shame on me". If someone becomes a repeat offender and continually disrespects you, then it's time to forgive, cut them out of your life and never forget.

This reminds me of my past and the friendly relationship I had with a neighbour of mine at school whom I socialised with on a regular basis. It was happenstance that we became friends. We were of similar age, and we happened to be neighbours, so naturally enough we were in each other's company a lot. Other than this we didn't have much in common. However, it is only upon reflection on this relationship that I understand the many instances of disrespect I choose to overlook which was ultimately to my detriment. Now that I am older, I have distanced myself from him. However, my self-esteem and self-image continue to suffer. It is because of such experiences that I have come to realise that it is ok to stand up for yourself when the situation warrants it. I don't condone violence, but if someone is violent towards you, self-defence is acceptable. Notwithstanding this, I have also come to understand the power of words and the effect they can have. It is up to you to decide whether you want to lift people up or put them down.

Finally, forgiveness is not easy, however one thing that I keep in mind is that you must look at the perpetrator as an imperfect human. This concept makes forgiveness and easier endeavour. At the end of the day no human is perfect, and forgiveness becomes easier when you realise that the perpetrator has likely suffered from injustices too.

Task B: Essay Sample 31
Comment Set P

We all want to seem strong in this world. It is a tough world after all, full of hierarchy and domination. As such, forgiveness for wrongs done to us may seem weak and foolish. However, it is really an act of strength to forgive. It is also wise to do so given the context of all the wrongs we have done ourselves. As such, although it may seem weak and foolish to forgive, it is really strong and wise to do so.

It may seem like a weak and foolish act to forgive someone. This world we live in is such a harsh world, full of hierarchical mindsets and acts of domination over others. As such, it is understandable that people would want to appear strong and powerful. Therefore, to forgive someone may seem like we are giving in to our wrong-doers. It may signal that we are weak. Consequently, in the tough world we live in, it would seem like a foolish act. However, it is really being strong and wise to forgive. To go against the grain of societal opinion is a tough thing to do. It requires bravery, determination and grit. Furthermore, to forego the hurt that someone has done to you requires a level of emotional fortitude and maturity. Therefore, it demonstrates strength to forgive someone. Furthermore, it is wise, rather than foolish, to forgive.

There are a multitude of wrongs we have committed during our own lives. We may have cheated, lied, and hurt others' feelings. Indeed, some of the trespasses we have committed ourselves in the past may have been worse than that which was committed against us. This is illustrated in the parable Christ gave concerning the servant who owed several hundred talents of silver to a king, and who was forgiven his debt. However, shortly after, the same servant found a friend who owned him just a little money, and refused to forgive that debt. In the parable, the king then learnt of the servant's actions, and was very angry with him and threw him into debtor's jail. Such a parable was meant to illustrate how God had forgiven us for our grave and soul-damning sins. Therefore, whatever trespasses our neighbours have committed against us, we are meant to forgive, or else God would be wroth with us. As such, it is both a strong and a wise thing to forgive. Granted, it is not necessary to hug and kiss our perpetrators, or even to forget what they did to us. Indeed, some things that others have done to us may have been quite damaging and traumatic. Rather, forgiveness is simply relinquishing the debt you may hold over others. In other words, forgiveness is relinquishing feelings of revenge or desires of punishment upon one's perpetrators. Besides, punishment will come upon one's wrong doers, whether in this life or the next. It is not necessary for us to take responsibility for it. As such, holding onto grievances and unforgiveness would simply add stress to our lives.

In conclusion, although it may seem weak and foolish to forgive, it is actually strong, wise and stress-relieving to do so. Everyone wants to appear strong in this tough world we live in. In this regards, we may think we should not forgive others for the wrongs they may have done us. It would seem like a weak and, consequently, a foolish act. However, it takes bravery to act otherwise. Furthermore, there are a multitude of trespasses we have committed ourselves, some even graver. By not forgiving others for their trespasses against us, we may risk the ire of those who have already forgiven us for our graver wrongdoings. In addition, by not forgiving we cling on to feelings of aggrievement. Therefore, it is strong, wise, and stress-relieving to forgive others.

Comment Set Q

Comment 1

Courage is a mean with regard to fear and confidence.

Aristotle

****

Comment 2

Courage is of the heart by derivation, And great it is. But fear is of the soul.

Robert Frost

****

Comment 3

Courage doesn't always roar. Sometimes courage is the little voice at the end of the day that says I'll try again tomorrow.

Mary Anne Radmacher

****

Comment 4

Courage is being scared to death— and saddling up anyway.

John Wayne

****

Comment 5

Courage is grace under pressure

Ernest Hemingway

Task B: Essay Sample 32
Comment Set Q

When I was a child, one of my favourite films was the 'Lion King'. I would watch it over and over, never tiring of the musical numbers or watching the same storyline unfold each time. A part of the film which always stayed with me was when Mufasa saved his son, from the Hyenas. He chastised Simba, saying "being brave doesn't mean you go looking for trouble". At the time, I was far more interested in screaming, 'the circle of life' at the top of my lungs, than trying to unpack what this meant. But now, as I read the comments above, I am reminded of my favourite childhood film. I think now, what Mufasa meant, was that being courageous means responding to situations which are worthy of that fear, rather than seeking out danger or fear to prove courageousness in a reckless manner. I believe this parallels Aristotle's comment that "courage is a mean with regard to fear and confidence". By describing courage as the "mean" between fear and confidence, I think Aristotle means to tell us that courage is found at the point of equilibrium between two extremes. Courage is the thing that takes two vices; cowardice and recklessness, and brings them together to create a virtue. When a coward is faced with a daunting task, they turn and run from the face of danger or difficulty. Conversely, the reckless individual will blindly run into battle without thinking of the consequences. Between these two extremes is the brave, courageous individual. They remain composed and think about their options so as to defeat the danger bravely.

Hemingway makes a similar point to that of Aristotle when he proclaimed that courage was "grace under pressure". Like Aristotle, Hemingway suggests that courage is not quite like the movies or comic books make it out to be. It is not always about the strong, powerful superhero. Instead it can look much more plain. Like a swan gliding across the water with such elegance, we forget that beneath the surface, their legs must work very hard to push against the current. I think Hemingway's description of courage is similar to the image of the sawn. It isn't loud or boastful. It is calm and graceful. But, much like the legs of the swan under the water, there is a great deal of effort to be so graceful, it is just unseen. So, whilst the heroes, that authors love to tell us about in stories are more often thought of as being courageous and brave, we are wrong to make this generalisation. Courage is instead found in the most unassuming of places. Aristotle's definition of courage tells us that it is not brash action that makes a person courageous. Nor is it inaction. It is a composed, graceful state wherein the individual has taken into account all aspects of the danger in order to choose the appropriate action. If we imagine the swan as being the balance of the two vices we can further explain both Hemingway and Aristotle's idea. If the swan was to be a coward and simply give up fighting against the current, no longer moving its legs, then it would only move backwards. It would regress. However, if the swan used all of its energy, flapped its wings, and moved its legs with ferocious power, then it would tire and eventually meet the same fate as the coward. But, if the sawn were to be courageous, then it would swim enough to continue moving forward, but not too much to exhaust itself. It would find the balance between the two. The result would be the swan we know to admire, the graceful, elegant animal that seemingly moves along the water with ease.

John Wayne tells us that courage is about "being scared to death – but saddling up anyway". Although this seems like it would counteract Aristotle and Hemingway's idea of courage. I actually think it agrees with them both. You see, the important thing to note is that Wayne tells us that we saddle up anyway despite being scared. Scared is really the key word here because it tells us that Wayne also believes that being courageous requires you to understand and respect fear. If one were reckless and free from any fear of consequence, they would act in a blind and uncalculated manner. The point they all make is that we must understand that something is scary or dangerous in order to act bravely or courageously and we must hold on to a small piece of recklessness in order to overcome that fear and "saddle up".

As a child, watching the Lion King, I did not take into account the complexities of Mufasa's teaching. However, it always stayed with me and it is now, as an adult that I understand what he meant. We must choose our battles wisely and accept that fear is inevitable. In addition, we must know when to walk away and not act in a thoughtless manner. Throughout my life I have unknowingly followed Mufasa's advice, from when I was a small child, getting back up on my bike after I had fallen, but the next with knee guards, to this present day. I am thankful for what I learned about courage, as it has allowed me to live my life with joy and pleasure. The worst thing that we should be afraid of is fear itself because what could be more terrifying than getting to the end of your life and realising that you were a swan who gave up swimming?

Comment Set R

Comment 1

Where you will sit when you are old shows where you stood in youth.

****

Comment 2

You are only young once, but you can stay immature indefinitely.

Ogden Nash

****

Comment 3

Don't let anyone think little of you because you are young.

****

Comment 4

Youth is a phase that happens once in your life, but it is also a spark that you can carry in your heart forever.

Task B: Essay Sample 33
Comment Set R

Dear reader,

This essay examines the effects of early childhood abuse and neglect. Please be aware of this if these topics affect you.

In saying that "where you will sit when you are old shows where you stood in youth", Comment 1 is commenting on the permanence of our childhood experiences. It seems likely that Comment 1 is specifically alluding to socioeconomic status ("where you stood"/"where you will sit"). However, the statement can be applied more generally, to argue that what we experience during childhood has an irreversible effect on every stage of the lifespan following it. Oftentimes, these experiences are character-building and form a stable foundation with which we can use to navigate the rest of our lives – right through adulthood and into old age. At other times, these experiences are catastrophic (for example, childhood abuse and neglect) and can result in permanent social, emotional, or cognitive deficits.

Perhaps the most well-documented case of severe childhood abuse and neglect causing permanent harm through to adulthood and old age is the case study of "Genie". Genie was 11 years old when she was discovered by social workers in her parent's garage, strapped to a potty chair and unable to interact with her environment. She was fed meals through a slot in the garage door. She was unable to communicate verbally with her family – if her siblings made any attempt to speak with Genie, they themselves were punished severely. She had never learned to walk, talk, or socialise. Upon her discovery, Genie was immediately placed into therapy and studied extensively until her old age. She eventually learned to walk, although she never learned to speak full sentences or interact appropriately with others. Genie's case is now examined in most introductory psychology classes to demonstrate with painful clarity the time-sensitive nature of several essential cognitive functions, including language.

It is vital to discuss and examine Genie's story, as it serves as a striking example of how vulnerable we are as children to permanent change (whether it be positive or negative). In youth (particularly in very early childhood), we must achieve certain milestones (such as language acquisition) before it is too late – otherwise these milestones may never be overcome. This time-sensitive nature of childhood is alluded to in several of the stimulus quotes ("you are only young once"/"youth is a phase that happens once in your life"). Although the tone in these quotes is wistful (and not cautionary), they are statements of fact. Our childhood experiences only occur once, and they permanently affect our behaviour and well-being. This remains true even if we accept that Comment 1 is referring solely to socioeconomic status in childhood vs. adulthood – a mountain of evidence demonstrates that low socioeconomic status has long-lasting effects on cognition and behaviour.

Ultimately, the case study of Genie is an extreme example of how our childhood experiences affect us permanently. I chose to discuss Genie's case (despite the generally playful or sentimental undertones of the stimulus quotes), because, in my opinion, many people underestimate the long-lasting (and often permanent) effects of early childhood experiences. In my opinion, it is indeed true that "where you will sit when you are old shows where you stood in youth".

Task B: Essay Sample 34
Comment Set R

Age is just a number

Youth are often tagged as immature, lacking knowledge and wisdom, living in blissful ignorance with complete disregard for what is happening around them. But this couldn't be further from the truth. A lot of the time young people can be more compassionate, open minded and tolerant. Having not yet had their ideologies and opinions shaped by the strong political and social-cultural prejudices that dominate the media and the lives of adults, young people can be more powerful in influencing change.

It still surprises me to think of the impact I have been able to have on my grandpa. Having always sat him on a pedestal, believing him to have all the answers I never thought that at a mere 14-year-old I would be able to influence him to make changes. During the lead up to my 14 th birthday I decided that rather than receiving than keeping any presents I received for myself I would instead donate them to a child in need. Looking around at my cupboards that were overflowing, all the books that that sat in the corner because I had no room on my shelves. I didn't need anything else; I didn't want anything else, I just wanted to share the happiness that I would have gotten from the gifts with a child living in poverty. In my absolute determination wrote out quite wordy emails to all my family and friends explaining what I was going to do. My grandpa was shocked, at 14 he would never have given up getting the newest toy on his birthday. In fact, he was so moved by my desire to help others that he himself decided to donate to World Vision and sponsor a child in Africa to help improve their lives. At as young as 14 I was able to open the mind of my grandpa and influence him into donating (and he still does) and contributing to the fight to end poverty.

And while my personal experience may not be quite the ground-breaking change you were hoping for plenty of youth are continuing to make monumental changes across the globe for example Greta Thunberg her climate change movement, Malala Yousafzai and her fight for woman's education and Chanel Contos and her fight for consent education. All three of these women have been able to single handily inspire millions to join the fight for equality, safety, and environmental sustainability. Such young voices have been able to challenge world leaders and force changes in legislation inspiring millions. Greta has now inspired countries to make changes to their climate change policies, Chanel has changed the face of consent education in Australia and Malala has won a Nobel Peace Prize for her work for women's education.

So next time someone tells you that you're too young to make a difference, prove them wrong. Age is just a number.

Task B: Essay Sample 35
Comment Set R

A Timeless Tale

My mother was someone who truly influenced me to become an avid reader from a very young age, given to the fact that she herself was quite the lover of books. From introducing me to this new chapter of my life, I began to see a world of opportunities and imagination from words and letters inscribed within the pages of paperbacks and hardcovers. From Little House on the Prairie by Laura Ingalls Wilder, to all seven books of Harry Potter by J.K. Rowling, to Sir Arthur Conan Doyle's infamous Sherlock Holmes, I was besotted by these tales.

As I grew older, my love of books did not shrivel and die but grew older with me. I felt a sort of spark within me whenever I read books, as if it reminded me of all the feelings and wonders I had when I was a young girl, and it was this feeling that compelled me to read even more. I suppose it was this desire and passion for books that sort of defined my youth, as books for me were something that was timeless and ageless. If I picked up The Hunger Games and read it now, I would have the same feeling, that little flutter or spark in my heart, as I did when I was a twelve-year-old girl experiencing Katniss Everdeen's harsh new world for the first time.

Needless to say, going into high-school, I was met with a lot of questionable glances. I was getting older, yes, and my place in society was becoming little by little clearer to me. I had responsibilities, of course. I should not spend so much time buried away in books, as I should have been drowning in textbooks in science and French conjugation flashcards to ensure I graduate high-school with flying colours. I grew up in a very judgemental and competitive Sri-Lankan community in Australia, so of course I was met with a lot of side-eyes and wrinkled eyebrows as aunties and uncles would glance at this eighteen-year-old girl refusing to socialize because J.K. Rowling's world was much more interesting than a boring old dinner party.

Now here was the question-when was it too old to stop reading, or was reading a merely a pastime of the youth. It was a strange and funny thing, because the older I got, the more weight the world seemed to weigh on my shoulders. As one gets older, one begins to question whether if everything in life really feels like a chore. Were things you used to love as child seem more like you are ticking off something in a to-do list, weary and tired for the day in which you have to come back and do it again? It was like youth was a candle, and the older you grow up, the dimmer and less significant it got, until that bright light will eventually die away and you are left with nothing that made you happier as a child.

I believe that I would blame this phenomenon on the stresses of adult-life and the uncertainty it may bring. People begin to put expectations on you, society claims to know where you should be and what you should be doing once you turn sixteen, eighteen, twenty-one. Immaturity and childhood wonder are looked down upon, and its place you are filed away into a place that others have deemed right for you.

This was exactly what happened to me as I entered university. The stresses of high-school life and a sudden thrust into the adult world made me feel like my light was dimmed too fast, and the weight on my shoulder was no longer by school back-pack, but one that consisted of worrying about employment and stresses of life, or more so not knowing how to deal with such anxieties. It became hard for me to remember what true happiness was like, the joy of being immature due to the sudden pace in which I was forced to mature. I no longer felt like a child, and I no longer felt like reading. That was the saddest of all the parts.

I believe all those years of emptiness and anxiety was because of what I believed a true adult should live like-with responsibilities and a striving path for success. Sure, I was successful, but the little spark in my heart was gone. Instead, I felt myself spiralling into a dark sea of anxiety, in which I found myself worrying days on end about the smallest of inconveniences. I was confused as well as uncomfortable, as I felt as if I did not belong in this newer, more mature body of mine that I was somehow supposed to live and morph into for the rest of my life. They say that adulthood is like a new phase in life, like a baby caterpillar turning into a breathtakingly beautiful butterfly. Well, to say the truth, I sort of felt like the butterfly but without the pretty colours. More like a moth, really. Maybe in my heart I was still that little caterpillar.

A few years went by and on one of my birthdays, my mother gifted me with something quite special. It was a novel, which took me by surprise as I was quite certain that she knew that I have not read since high school, which was a very long time ago. My mother had a knowing look in her eyes, as if she was imploring me to trust her. So, I did, and I flipped open the first page of Jane Austen's Pride and Prejudice, and instantly fell in love with the world of Elizabeth Bennett and Mr. Darcy. I felt excited, exhilarated, giddy, and to tell you the truth, I felt free. I felt free in the sense that I was unshackled from my responsibilities as an adult, and not once did I feel guilty for taking some time for myself and dwelling in the luxuries of my youth that I had enjoyed so many times.

It was a strange, sudden, beautiful realisation, to be reminded that growing old and becoming and adult does not mean you should abandon your childhood loves and follies simply because society has unattainable standards. Youth is a precious time and for me it was defined by books and novels and those magical, magical worlds built words upon words. To others, it may be different, but the message is still the same. As the saying goes, "Youth is a phase that happens once in your life, but it is also a spark that you can carry in your heart forever." You should never give up what defines your youth, because that is your butterfly moment.

Comment Set S

Comment 1

Being a pessimist has its merit: you are constantly taking precautions.

****

Comment 2

It doesn't hurt to be optimistic. You can always try again.

****

Comment 3

We can look at rosebushes having thorns or thorn bushes having roses.

****

Comment 4

Some people see the glass half full. Others see it half empty. I see a glass that's twice as big as it needs to be.

George Carlin

Task B: Essay Sample 36
Comment Set S

(Title choices: 1.The Descent into Hell, 2. Carpe Diem, 3. Paradise Lost)

Although changing one's perspectives may help one deal with many of life's problems, there may be limitations to how much one can change as an individual. Although people face seemingly tough situations, they may feel a lot better if they compared their current situation with their past situations in life, or with other people in worst circumstances around the world. However, such changes of one's individual perspectives may have its limits, particularly in tough situations where state oppression is involved. Despite this, by going a step further and by reconsidering one's expectations of life on earth, this may help one avoid disappointment.

Having a change in perspective may help to resolve many of one's life's problems. Oftentimes, we think the problems of life are insurmountable and about how terrible our situations are. However, our feelings about our current situations may change if we consider past difficulties we have surmounted or if we consider greater difficulties that other people around the world may be experiencing. For example, I may be stressed and depressed about my lack of career and position in society at my age, as well as my stagnant financial situation. However, my perspectives and feelings may change if I consider the refugees stuck in immigration detention in Australia or, indeed, the people around the world stuck in war zones. Indeed, comparing myself to the people in those situations, my position may actually feel quite okay. The problems I seem to face may pale in comparison, and I may feel more thankful for the freedoms and privileges I enjoy. Indeed, as some have said, I may now view life as a rose, and the relatively few problems I face as minor thorns around its stem. In this regard, methods such as Cognitive Behavioural Therapy can assist people to think through their problems methodically and to rank and compare them to see if they are really that bad. Such strategies may be beneficial and should be considered by many people in the first instance to help them cope with the feelings they are experiencing about their life's problems.

However, there may be limitations to how much one can improve by simply changing their individual perspectives. Indeed, there are certain problems that no matter how hard one tries, they are difficult to will away or to be thought of in a more positive light. For example, consider if you are the person who is the refugee stuck in immigration limbo. If you have been detained for more than ten years, eating awful food and living in cramped and paltry conditions, with no legal avenue to settle in Australia, and a government in your home country waiting to execute you on your return, who else would you compare yourself too? Indeed, it may seem like a neo-Liberal myth that the individual has power and can do anything in life, so long as they tried hard enough. However, when one is on the wrong side of state oppression, it would instead feel like the individual is powerless and cannot do anything no matter how hard they tried. As such, there may be a limitation to how much an individual can change by trying to change their own individual perceptions. Despite this, one could be thankful that one is still alive and not currently in an active war zone. But, is that asking too little of life? Perhaps, like Carlin, we may answer no, it is not asking too little of life. Rather than considering whether our life is half empty, or half full, we may say it is just about right if we just lowered our expectations of it. That is to say, what many have been asking of life on this earth has been too much and if they just lowered their expectations, they would not be so disappointed.

In conclusion, although changing one's perspectives on life can make one feel better, there are limitations to how much this can help, though perhaps not so if one were to descend even lower. Having a change in individual perspective can help one deal with many of life's problems. By considering past difficulties, or by considering people in worst situations, one can feel a lot better about one's current situations. However, such strategies can have their limitations. In the context where one is already in one of the worst situations on the planet, such as a powerless subject under state oppression, it is difficult to see the positives in life. In spite of this, by going a step further down and by reconsidering the purpose, and worth, of an individual's life on earth, one may even breach this level in one's self-concept and, thus, avoid disappointment.

Comment Set T

Comment 1

...inside every old person is a young person wondering what happened.

Terry Pratchett, Moving Pictures

****

Comment 2

I am incapable of conceiving infinity, and yet I do not accept finity. I want this adventure that is the context of my life to go on without end.

Simone de Beauvoir, La Vieillesse

****

Comment 3

Many things can prolong your life, but only wisdom can save it.

Neel Burton

****

Comment 4

I was brought up to respect my elders, so now I don't have to respect anybody.

Pablo Picasso

****

Comment 5

Youth is a dream, a form of chemical madness.

George Burns

Task B: Essay Sample 37
Comment Set T

"Youth is a dream, a form of chemical madness" (George Burns). The saturated dream-like picture of youth, where young adults are thrown into a world of opportunity and exploration and everything is exciting and free for their taking. Older generations often refer to the youth as selfish and lazy, as they appear to lack discipline and responsibilities when compared to older adults. Since the beginning of history, the elderly have been respected for their wisdom as a result of life experience, which gives them life insights that younger people may lack. In my life, I have often looked to the elderly for guidance on how to live a better life.

"Young, Wild, and Free". The time when young people finish school and are unleashed into the world feels like years of summer, with endless travel, parties, and music. They mainly seek the hedonic pleasures of life, often under the justification of needing to have fun while they're young, and to "find themselves". What inevitably follows is the middle age, which Doris Day referred to as "youth without levity, and age without decay". This is when the dull, robot-like 9-5 working routines come into effect for most, where days consist mostly of work, food, and sleep. Many sacrifice their passions for their perceived duties, and these days drag on into old age.

Author and hospice nurse Bronnie Ware asked elderly in palliative care to write down what they regretted the most, a few weeks before they passed away. The number one regret most people had was not having had the courage to live a life true to themselves and instead doing what was expected of them. The second biggest regret was working so hard, noting the bitterness and resentment they held as a result. Lastly, they wished they had let themselves be happier.

These comments of the elderly have encouraged me to reflect on my own life throughout the years. I have spent the majority of my life completing my duties as a mother, wife, and worker. This usually meant a lack of time and often money for travel and parties, and over the time my childhood dreams faded and were forgotten. As Terry Pratchett so precisely put it: "Inside every old person is a young person wondering what happened". What would my life have looked like if I followed my "chemical madness" of young thoughts and dreams every step of the way? What person would I have become?

I remember being young and just packing up to move to Germany in my early 20's, without any future plans or a care in the world. Now, I judge my daughter when she tries to do the same for being irresponsible in fears of her jeopardising her future. But the more I become aware of this, the more I seek my child self for guidance. I am proud to have accomplished everything I have, and perhaps I would not be as successful in my life and career had I just followed that chemical madness. I believe, as with everything there needs to be a balance. I work hard and make sacrifices for the things that are important, but I also need my inner child to bring back the fun and colour into life.

Comment Set U

Comment 1

The worst loneliness is not to be comfortable with yourself.

Mark Twain

****

Comment 2

Solitude is the profoundest fact of the human condition. Man is the only being who knows he is alone.

Octavio Paz

****

Comment 3

Loneliness is a barrier that prevents one from uniting with the inner self.

Carl Rogers

****

Comment 4

At the innermost core of all loneliness is a deep and powerful yearning for union with one's lost self.

Brendan Francis

****

Comment 5

To dare to live alone is the rarest courage; since there are many who had rather meet their bitterest enemy in the field, than their own hearts in their closet.

Charles Caleb Colton

Task B: Essay Sample 38
Comment Set U

In my childhood, I used to think that loneliness is just being alone, but that view has since changed. Prominent psychological research has described loneliness as lack of connection. Often this has been interpreted as lack of social connection. This essay attempts to detail how loneliness can be interpreted in two primary forms: lack of connection with others, and lack of connection with oneself, with lack of self-connection being particularly detrimental.

Lack of connection with others stimulates loneliness. Consider the case of me in middle school. After a tumultuous move from another country and the social blunder of mispronouncing a classmate's name, I was left alone and separated from my peers. This is the primary interpretation of loneliness. Even though I wanted to have friends to sit with at lunch, I didn't, and hence I felt lonely. This view of loneliness as a social phenomenon is a reasonable one to hold as human beings are social beings, with many psychological studies citing that socialisation is one the key regulating factors for our emotions. Indeed, a psychological research study even found that loneliness is "catching" and can spread from social network to social network, thus cementing loneliness as rooted in social connection. However, this interpretation would suggest that the antidote for loneliness is just making social connections. This may not always be true.

Purely making social connections does not "solve" loneliness. As detailed above, middle school for me was a very isolating experience. However, eventually, I did manage to make a few friends. Whilst this did indeed resolve my issue of where I was going to sit at lunch, surprisingly I didn't feel that much happier. What I've learnt from this experience is that it is simply not enough to make more social connections to "fix" loneliness. When hanging out with my new friends, the activities we took part in gave me no real happiness as this was not what I truly wanted, hence I was lonely even when I was with other people. The aspect of my happiness which depended on my being true to myself was still unfulfilled, which still kept me lonely. Hence, loneliness can only be truly solved when your actions are aligned with your heart.

Living in accordance with your inner self can curb loneliness. Consider me during the COVID-19 pandemic. Despite people reporting feeling lonely at record highs due to lack of social connection, surprisingly I felt okay. Despite the fact that my social connections were not well nurtured during quarantine periods, my actions were aligned to who I truly was. Whereas before I forced myself to participate in activities that were meaningless to me, now, the ceasure of those activities meant that I took the time to figure out what made me really happy and did those things. Hence, loneliness is not always about social connection, but also about uniting with your inner self.

In sum, loneliness can be interpreted in two primary ways. Whilst popularly loneliness is simply the absence of other people detrimentally impacting us due to our social nature, the presence of others does not necessarily cure our loneliness. The essence of curing loneliness stems from connecting with your true self and valuing those inner desires. Hence, the most valuable thing we can do in recovering from loneliness is not only to surround ourselves with people, but to also listen to our hearts.

Task B: Essay Sample 39
Comment Set U

Loneliness is a worst feeling of a mankind. It does not let our innersoles get involved in any situation. Eventhough, we are physically surrounded by many people, we are feeling lonely because our state of mind is not accompanying our physical situation and people surrounding us. I believe that there is a great difference between loneliness and being alone. Loneliness deteriorates one's mental condition whereas being alone is a positive attitude towards life.

I would like to share one of my incidents. I have always dreamt to be a doctor. And for that I have had worked my ass off during my high school days. I still remember the feeling of looking at my year 12 results. It was a worst feeling. It felt like my surrounding was shaking when I realised that I missed out by two points from getting into medicine school. I soaked my pillow with tears. I was surrounded by my family and friends, but all I was thinking about was my results and my future. All the thoughts in my mind were fighting a battle. I was coming up all kind of weird feelings. Feeling of fear, feeling of sadness, feeling of getting broke. People surrounding me were trying to motivate me, encourage me by saying that it was not an end, but it was just me trapped in a circle of loneliness that did not want to get involved in those nonsensical talks. I was feeling that people surround me were not understanding me as they never have been through such situation. Time heals everything. Here, I am, got my courage back and figured out the other way of getting into medical school.

However, being alone is a positive attitude that one carries. As said by Charles Caleb Colton, "To dare to live alone is the rarest courage; since there are many who had rather meet their bitterest enemy in the field, than their own hearts in their closet". Being alone, gives an opportunity to see innersoles and reflect towards ourselves. I always prefer to go for an evening walk by myself. This gives me time for myself. I think about my present life and my career. I can get chance about what I really want to pursue in my life and the way of achieving that. Being alone helps me to reflect on my perspective and purpose of life.

In conclusion, loneliness is something that person feels, even though he is surrounded by a group of people. Person feels lonely, when people surrounding him is not understanding or they are not considerate about his perspective towards situation. Whereas, being alone is essential and fosters one to achieve great things in life.

Comment Set V

Comment 1

People are trapped in history and history is trapped in them.

****

Comment 2

History is a set of lies agreed upon.

****

Comment 3

Civilization is a movement and not a condition, a voyage and not a harbour.

****

Comment 4

With malice towards none, with charity for all, with firmness in the right, as God gives us to see the right, let us finish the work we are in, to bind up the nation's wounds.

Task B: Essay Sample 40
Comment Set V

It is true that some people are trapped in history and history is trapped in them. History is important as the lessons learned from history can be useful to make our present and future better however getting trapped in history isn't a good idea as it curbs both the growth and the possibility of a change. Hence, it is important for people to realize that one can only seek inspiration from history and eventually one has to advance in life.

People are trapped in history which can curb the growth of the individual. Ideally individuals should remember the lessons from history and then move on to adapt to a new future. However, people struggle to achieve that balance. It is important to investigate the reason behind people being trapped in history. People sometimes are unable to advance in life due to the fear of losing the emotional ties that they might have with a person or a thing. Some people struggle, because they cannot accept the reality and hence cannot advance in life. This can be explained by the 5 stages of grief including denial, anger, bargaining, depression, and acceptance. Some people probably get trapped in the first four stages which don't allow them to reach the stage of acceptance. The dormancy doesn't allow an individual to adapt to a changing future which is supposed to bring growth and prosperity. This is problematic as everyone want to progress in their life to achieve fulfillment and happiness.

To counter this, it is vital for people to understand that one can advance in life by not moving on but moving forward with history. Human beings are evolutionally emotional beings that have to deal with multiple emotions. In order to transcend the different stages mentioned above, it is important to identify, acknowledge, and investigate the origins of the different emotions. This will eventually allow them to take an action and advance in life. For example, a person who has lost a loved one has to spend time in the five stages mentioned above and analyse the emotions that person experiences during that time. This will eventually allow them to move forward in life with the memories of the loved one in their heart. It is also important to not ignore the past events as history teaches us important lessons. The experiences serve as a reminder of how we should be leading our life. For example, we have learned from past that religious differences have led to the partition of a country like India to India and Pakistan. As a result of this, we now believe in secularism which has separated religion from governmental affairs. Hence, we should always keep our past close to our heart but also ensure that we don't get trapped in it.

History teaches us important lessons about life that allows us to make informed decisions in the present. Hence, it is important to keep the past events close to our heart. However, it is equally important to move forward with history to allow for growth and prosperity to take place.

Looking for more? No problemo! More sample, model essays can be found online in your gamsat-prep.com account.

If you give a sincere effort and really develop content for WC 4.5.1, 4.5.2, 4.6.1, 4.6.2 and 4.11, then in the days and hours leading up to the real GAMSAT, revising that content will be one of your most valuable tools to optimise your Written Communication GAMSAT score. Good luck!